Clinical Ethics

CLINICAL ETHICS

An Invitation to Healing Professionals

William dePender
&
Wanda Ikeda-Chandler

PRAEGER

New York
Westport, Connecticut
London

R724
D458
1990

Library of Congress Cataloging-in-Publication Data

dePender, William.
  Clinical ethics : an invitation to healing professionals / William
dePender, Wanda Ikeda-Chandler.
    p.   cm.
  Includes bibliographical references.
  ISBN 0–275–93437–3 (alk. paper)
    1. Medical ethics.   2. Medical care—Moral and ethical aspects.
I. Ikeda-Chandler, Wanda.   II. Title.
[DNLM: 1. Ethics, Medical.   W   50   D419c]
R724.D458   1990
174'.2—dc20   89–16224

Library of Congress Catalog Card Number: 89–16224
ISBN: 0–275–93437–3

First published in 1990

Praeger Publishers, One Madison Avenue, New York, NY 10010
A division of Greenwood Press, Inc.

Printed in the United States of America

The paper used in this book complies with the
Permanent Paper Standard issued by the National
Information Standards Organization (Z39.48–1984).

10 9 8 7 6 5 4 3 2 1

Contents

Introduction   vii

1 The Backdrop   1

2 The Confusion about Ethics   15

3 Ethics and the Health Sciences   27

4 The Vocabulary   41

5 The Problems and Issues   51

6 Five Traditional Approaches   63

7 The Personalist Approach   75

8 Putting Theory into Practice   93

9 Social Ethics (Politics)   105

Conclusion   119

Appendix: Discussion of the Case Examples   125

Bibliography   139

Index   141

Introduction

This is an ethics book for nonethicists. It's for those who want to learn more about ethics, but aren't sure where to begin. It presumes an orientation toward helping people who are ill, rather than a background in philosophical theory.

The newcomer to ethics will learn what ethics is about, and what ethics has to offer the healing professional. The vocabulary of ethics is introduced in a manageable way, and the most commonly used ethical theories are presented and discussed. Those who already have a working knowledge of ethics will find a new approach to ethical theory offered, one that the authors believe can make our practical use of ethics more effective and reliable. By the end of the book, the reader will have the tools to use ethical reasoning to work toward meaningful and reproducible answers to difficult ethical problems.

There's a fundamental question, though, that needs to be answered before we proceed. Is it really worthwhile for the "average" health care professional to spend time learning more about ethics? Indeed, some still believe that ethics is too difficult a topic for nonphilosophers. Of course, when ethical theory is presented in a complicated or confusing way, this is true—but ethics isn't *necessarily* difficult.

Some maintain that spending time on ethics distracts us from more important matters of patient care—that it's a waste of time. Hardly. Reflecting on what we're doing, on what it all means, can put organization into our efforts. It can minimize our false starts and backtracking. It can make our professional careers more fluid and effective. In the long run, thinking about what we're doing saves time, it doesn't waste it.

Still, why not leave ethics to philosophers? Why not let them do their job, and profit from their results? The best reason is that we have something indispensable to offer. Even though philosophers work very deeply with ideas, healers have the unique, practical experience of making important decisions with those who are ill. In fact, healers deal with ethical problems every day, whether they recognize it or not. They have more experience in dealing with difficult ethical questions than nearly anyone in our society. They engage difficult human problems, they make decisions, and they stand by them.

The bottom line is this: excellent decisions *are* made—every day—as they've been made for generations by excellent healers who've delivered excellent health care. It is this heritage that qualifies healers to get involved with building a more solid foundation for health care ethics.

Are nurses, physical therapists, physicians, and social workers qualified to "do" ethics? Even if they never took a philosophy course in college? Even if they never struggled through a single, sedating chapter of Kant or Aristotle? Yes, they are. They are uniquely qualified by their experience, and by their lifelong commitment to doing the right thing. They're qualified because they have first-hand knowledge of the matters of life and death, human values, and human needs.

But isn't health care ethics just a frill, a side dish to the main course? No it isn't. It's a necessary ingredient. Ethics isn't an optional extra to quality healing, it's standard equipment. Patients count on their healers to do what's best for them. They rely on healing professionals to handle a life crisis as if it were an everyday event. This is part of what makes it a privilege to be a healer—and it's also part of what makes it so difficult. Healers are people too. This kind of heavy responsibility can be difficult to live with.

This may be one of the most important reasons for perfecting our ethical skills: we do it for ourselves. We do it so that we can feel better about what we do for a living, so that we can go to work with the confidence that we're capable of making a real contribution. We do it so that we can find success even in situations where our technological wonders leave us high and dry.

Is ethics more than just daydreaming? Does ethical discussion really make a difference? It does. Putting our thoughts and insights out into the open helps us clarify and refine them. It measures our ideas against the reflections of others, and it solidifies the best of all those ideas. It does make a difference if we're listening and thinking. But sharing our ideas demands that we speak up.

Perhaps this is the biggest drawback to a public involvement with ethical thinking. Maybe we won't sound quite as brilliant as we'd like to sound. Maybe our ideas won't make sense, or will be just plain wrong. Who needs that? Actually, the risks are small, and the potential rewards great. The only way to find out what's going to happen is to give it a try.

So, the question isn't, "Should we, as healing professionals, be doing ethics?" We really can't avoid it. The real question is whether or not we should devote ourselves to building and refining our ethical skills. In this book we will make a strong case for bringing our ethical reflections out into the open.

Rather than being a simple introduction, then, this book is intended to be an invitation. Its goal is to encourage health care workers to "take the plunge," to become actively and openly involved in the pursuit of excellent ethical reasoning. This means orienting ourselves less toward standard treatments and more toward the best care that is humanly possible.

Chapter 1 highlights some of the modern issues that have renewed our society's interest in ethics. These issues provide the backdrop for our study of ethics. They include the personal and social concerns raised by our growing reliance on technology, our society's increasing malpractice problem, and the movement toward health care for profit. The questions, though, are just the start. As we proceed, we'll be focusing much more on answers.

Chapter 2 gives a definition of ethics that can help point us toward those answers. It looks more specifically at what ethics is, and what it isn't. Chapter 3 examines the goals of health care, and how ethics fits in with those goals.

The middle chapters (4 and 5) introduce the specialized vocabulary of ethics and discuss some common ethical issues.

Chapter 6 outlines several traditional theories that have been used to work toward answering these problems.

Chapter 7 offers another approach to ethical theory, one that is modeled closely after the traditions found in the healing arts. This approach fits more naturally with the orientation of the healer, rather than the academician. This is the personalist approach, and its influence is unavoidably present throughout the book.

Chapter 8 is frankly pragmatic, transporting ethical theory to the clinical setting. It offers a practical approach to getting started again when we feel as if things aren't working out, but we aren't sure why. Chapter 9 looks at social issues more directly, illustrating how ethics can help guide our society's future in a productive and meaningful way. As an appendix, there is a discussion of the case studies that are sprinkled throughout the book. The cases, of course, are real, and the appendix gives a brief narrative of their actual outcome as well as a short commentary.

Why spend time thinking about ethics at all? Why not just use that extra time to read another journal or even just vegetate in front of the television? Actually, there are plenty of good reasons to bring our interest in ethics into public view. In Chapter 1 we'll inventory some of the most urgent ones.

Clinical Ethics

1   The Backdrop

Not long ago, the word "ethics" hardly ever came up. When it did, it often meant that someone was about to lose a license, a job, or a lawsuit. Now, all of a sudden, health care ethics is a popular topic. There are conferences, committees, and books devoted to the subject. Is this just another fad? Or an academic hobby for a few enthusiasts? Will all this excitement over ethics be forgotten next year, or the year after that? Probably not. Too many people are growing interested in health care ethics for it to just fade away. People with very diverse backgrounds and points of view are starting to ask ethical questions.

Patients, concerned that their personal needs might not be met by an increasingly impersonal medical system, want their opinions heard. Nurses and physicians, regularly facing issues of life and death, are turning to ethics as a guide to better decision making. Even the courts, bogged down by unproductive conflict, are looking for better ways of expressing the values our society stands for.

The world is becoming more complicated with each passing year—and it's not likely to get simpler. We're surrounded by new technology, by social reform, and by communications that make the other side of the world seem like next door. Health care workers hardly think twice about feats that would have been utterly miraculous only a few decades ago. In a way, these changes are exciting, but in another way they can be terrifying.

We have more choices open to us than ever before, but we also have more confusion. In order to continue our progress, as individuals and as a society, we need a sense of direction.

Defining our goals, our values, is what ethics is about. That's why more and more people are getting interested in what ethics has to offer.

Many still see ethics as an intimidating subject. They think that ethics involves boring philosophical texts and dry, pointless arguments. Not so. Discovering and reflecting on our values can be stimulating, and it can be very practical. It can help us take charge of our lives. It can help us get more involved. It can renew our confidence in ourselves. Ethics doesn't have to be dull.

TECHNOLOGY: THE PERSONAL QUESTIONS

Case 1

Mrs. O is a seventy-six-year-old lady with multiple chronic medical problems. She has just been admitted to the hospital for yet another "tune-up." Unfortunately, her general condition seems to have deteriorated quite a bit in recent weeks. The consensus of the staff is that this will be her last admission.

You remember Mrs. O from previous hospitalizations. As her day nurse, you pick up a few not-so-subtle clues that she's frustrated by her failing health. She seems especially concerned about her code status. She's afraid that she will end her life tied to a variety of strange machines, squandering the savings that she had dreamt of leaving to her two children.

Her physician seems almost superstitiously reluctant to address the issue. The hospital chart continues to list her as "full code." Mrs. O is obviously anxious and troubled by the ambiguity of her situation. You feel you should become more visibly involved, but you're afraid that you'll be considered a troublemaker.

Just a couple of generations ago, there were no intensive care units (ICUs) and no "living wills." Mrs. O's kinds of concerns about death and dying simply didn't exist. Now they seem to be a fact of life. In simpler times, healers were plagued by the question, "What *can* we do for this patient?" Now, more and more often, we have to ask ourselves, "What *should* we do here?" In other words, now that we have more choices, we also have to decide which choices are really best. This new level of decision making is sort of an automatic "by-problem" of effective technology, and it can be much more demanding than simply picking a treatment from a book.

By developing new medical tools, we've opened important new doors for ourselves and for our patients, but we've also added complexity to our lives. This complexity has become a new problem in itself—a problem we can't solve with more technology. Nor can we make the problem go away by halting our scientific progress. Like Pandora, we can't unlearn what we already know.

We have "expensive care units," where the highest-tech is routine. In them, we help people survive enormous physical trials, intact and ready to continue their lives. But we sometimes find ourselves turning the process of dying into a macabre nightmare. People are afraid of long, painful deaths.

We have antibiotics that can overcome the most threatening infections. We keep nature at bay until physical strength returns. But we sometimes find ourselves playing dominoes in a cascade of losses that ultimately arrives nowhere. Watching these cases, people imagine themselves in a similar predicament, and they lose confidence.

We make resuscitation routine, almost habitual. It's easy, with intravenous (IV) fluids and drugs that correct each physiologic weakness. But our results aren't always what we wish they were, and people worry that painful procedures will be done *to* them rather than *for* them. They aren't comfortable with all these miracles.

Many of our patients, confronting the medical system, are like travelers in a faraway land, where the language and customs are foreign. Not having time to learn everything they need to know, they look for a guide, someone they can trust. Even fiercely independent patients can surprise their care-givers with the simple statement, "Do whatever you think is best." This charming sentiment can strike cold fear into the hearts of sensitive nurses and physicians.

These needs can't be shrugged off; they are legitimate and real. Unfortunately, what's best for one person may not be remotely right for another. The scientific model that calls for doing precisely the same thing each time simply won't work. So we need another model to guide us with these human problems, one that takes the human factor into account—that is, the ethical model.

Answering our important, nonscientific questions is the task of ethics; and that's partly why ethics is becoming an increasingly important topic. We have questions that can't be solved statistically—they can only be dealt with through a new and more thoughtful way of approaching life. Ethics is the name we give to a reflective consideration of our choices, our actions, and their results.

Many people have recently rediscovered the fact that there is an excellent time and place for stepping away from our medical machinery in favor of more old-fashioned ways of getting involved. But when and where and how? When do we make that final decision to turn off the IV fluids that sustain the helpless newborn? Where do we turn for help when our scientific bag of tricks is empty and our patient is dying? How do we carry difficult decisions through once we've made them, and how do we keep from getting exhausted in the process?

Should we operate on patients simply because we don't have anything else to offer? Should we run expensive tests looking for diseases we don't know how to treat? If we don't operate, if we don't run those tests, is there something else we could be doing, or should we just walk away?

Science deals only with quantities. As a society, we're coming to appreciate, again, that much of the process of healing revolves around qualities: relationships, responsibilities, mutual trust and openness, understanding. These are concepts that completely resist scientific definition, yet are critically important to the process of good medical decision making. So we turn to ethics. In the process, we don't have to turn away from technology, or anything else. We are simply trying to develop a side of ourselves that is capable of dealing with qualities, of recognizing human values as real and important. These new skills don't detract from our old ones, they add to them and make them even more effective.

Our new approach to technology is becoming more moderate and more mature. As our infatuation with technology dims, we find ourselves asking more permanent types of questions. "What are we really trying to accomplish?" "What does it all mean?" These aren't new questions—they've been asked over and over by philosophy. Ironically, it is our involvement with modern technology that is redirecting our attention toward these ancient issues.

TECHNOLOGY: THE SOCIAL QUESTIONS

Case 2

You are a resident on the trauma surgery team in a busy public hospital. One afternoon, a young man is wheeled into the emergency room with a gunshot wound to the chest. Cardiopulmonary resuscitation (CPR) is underway. Your team begins to work on him, and he seems to be responding. The operating room should be ready for him in about twenty minutes. The paramedics say that Mr. Y was shot by police officers at the scene of an attempted robbery, and that another person was also injured, apparently by Mr. Y.

A second ambulance arrives, this time bringing Mr. Y's purported victim. She is a woman in her mid-thirties, well-dressed, and she has a chest wound similar to Mr. Y's. She is also receiving CPR. You call for help, but you know that the backup team won't be available for at least thirty minutes. You also realize that it's unlikely your team will be able to save both victims. You wonder whom you should try to save.

Technology is a physical resource like any other. There never seems to be enough to go around. In the case of Mr. Y and his victim, there are only two people competing for the available technology; but on a larger scale, all of us are competing for what's new. In fact, the more we invent, the more we have to face the problem of short supply.

For example, suppose a powerful new scanner is invented. It can detect certain cancers a bit earlier, allowing more successful intervention. Experts predict that each machine could save fifty lives each year, but the cost of the equipment is staggering. Are we obligated to abandon our older technology in order to save those lives? Or should we abandon the new machine because we can't afford to make it available to everyone?

A third alternative, of course, is to make the use of the new machine available to anyone who can afford to pay the bill. Unfortunately, health care is very different from most other commodities—it saves lives. Can we allow it to be distributed in the same way as powerboats or televisions? How does that represent our supposed belief that "all men are created equal?"

Idealistic statements, though, won't solve our problem. Even if we could afford to provide everyone with the highest level of health care technology (which we can't), we still couldn't produce equipment fast enough to make it available to everyone before it, too, became obsolete. So we come full circle. Who will get the benefit of the latest developments, and who will have to settle for less? Which child will get the liver transplant, and which will be lost without a fight?

Is it society's responsibility to provide for our health care, or is that up to each of us as individuals? Is there some minimum level of care that each person is entitled to, or should we do everything we can for everybody? If we try to do too much for too many, will we cripple our ability to provide for our other important needs, such as education and housing?

Some of these questions become more confusing the more deeply we study them. Does everyone even *deserve* the same level of medical care? Does the smoker or the alcoholic have the same rights to our resources as the child with a congenital illness? Then again, does anyone really *choose* to be ill? Can any of us really judge the choices that others have made?

Once we start considering these difficult issues, it isn't long before we find ourselves confronting global issues as well. What about the less developed nations of the world? Are we somehow responsible to them as common children of a single planet? With the world becoming smaller each passing year, do our responsibilities to others grow? Then again, if we overextend our help to others, will we just drag ourselves down, without accomplishing a thing?

These aren't easy questions. A crystal ball would be nice; but being aware of the questions isn't enough. We have to get involved with finding answers. Even though many of these problems have come up recently, they aren't likely to resolve themselves spontaneously. Our most reasonable approach involves a thoughtful and cooperative discussion of these questions, sharing our thoughts about possible answers. When we take this approach we're "doing" ethics.

Of course, we could ignore these ethical questions, propelled by habit or expediency. Some might even suggest that such an approach is actually best. But, more and more, people want to take part in shaping the course of our society's future, and that's where ethics comes in. Of course, ethics can't guarantee our success, but it can offer a greater opportunity for success than blind chance.

Some might argue that these social issues should be left to judges and legislators. Most elected officials, though, would disagree. Referring to their "responsibilities to their constituencies," they're reminding us that they are the spokespersons of our society, but not the final architects of our society's values. That task belongs equally to us all.

So, paradoxically, the successes of technology are guiding us toward a renewed appreciation for the ancient philosophical discipline of ethics. Our continued scientific advances will probably make this need even more pressing as we continue into the future.

THE LAW

The topic of medical malpractice seems to evoke a certain morbid fascination in health care workers. We know good doctors who've been sued, and bad ones who haven't. Is there any logic to it? Sometimes the settlements and awards sound more like a lottery than a restitution. The entertainment value, though, fades when we stop to consider where that money ultimately comes from and, more soberingly, where it often goes.

Law and medicine have increasingly come head to head. Publicly, each profession maintains that it is "just doing its job," and that the causes of the malpractice problem lie elsewhere. More candidly, each would admit that there are complex internal problems that have helped foster the predicament in which we now find ourselves.

It seems ironic that, at a time when the medical field is able to do more than ever before, there clearly seems to be more consumer dissatisfaction than in the past. Some think that the lay public has simply been spoiled and is now making unreasonable demands. Not so. The problem is that the lay public is subtly aware that their more important human needs are frequently not being met.

Case 3

Mrs. F is twenty-two weeks along in her pregnancy when her labor prematurely begins. Dr. B examines her and finds her cervix to be dilated to nearly three centimeters. The membranes are hour-glassing. He begins her on ritodrine, and takes her to the delivery room to install a cerclage. During the procedure, the membranes rupture. Dr. B observes that he has done his very best, and goes home. Later that night the nonviable infant is delivered. The patient and her family seem less than satisfied.

Dr. A finds himself in an identical situation, and the medical outcome is the same. However, he calls the family together and spends some time coaxing them to share their deep feelings of loss. He also shares with them his own feelings of inadequacy and frustration. Their relationship with him now seems even more solid than before.

Dr. A seems to know something Dr. B doesn't. The loss of the baby isn't a completed event when the "specimen" has been sent to the lab. In fact, that may be just the beginning of the problem. Seeing things through can be as much a part of good care as being up to date on the latest techniques. There are some very practical issues here as well. When people are given the opportunity to work out their problems and differences together, they usually will. The drawback is that this can take time. The good news is that an hour at the bedside can be worth a week in the courtroom.

Conflict and litigation are often a by-product of suspicion. Suspicion grows when important concerns are ignored. Suspicion breeds fear. Fear increases the possibility of misunderstanding. And the cycle continues. This cycle breaks out into public view when legal action is taken, but the cycle itself isn't broken.

The courts may have the authority to decree an end to disputes, but they simply aren't the final mediators of understanding. In fact, the conflict that occurs in our legal system rarely fosters understanding at all—it more commonly breeds anger and resentment.

There are countless tips on how to avoid the headache of malpractice suits. Some say that scrupulous documentation is the key. Others say that ordering lots of tests will usually protect us. Still others say that nothing will help—the lawyers will "get us" no matter what.

In fact, the best approach to our current legal woes doesn't depend on more detailed consent forms, or more thorough paperwork to "cover ourselves." The real answer lies in more careful attention to the complete human needs of our patients. Ethics helps us deal with these problems ourselves, and, in so doing, defend ourselves and our patients from unproductive conflict.

More sophisticated scientific techniques won't solve our legal problems; they will probably just make them even worse. In fact, our infatuation with technology has been a major contributor to the problem. Of course, it isn't the technology itself that has weakened the patient-healer bond, but our fascination with it, to the exclusion of more important matters. Ethics can teach us to refocus our attention.

Because of widespread legal paranoia and the current emphasis on self-protective detail, we sometimes find ourselves wondering, "Do these people (patients) expect us to be *perfect?*" Few of us can function effectively or comfortably in such an atmosphere. But it isn't perfection that patients demand, it's reasonable competence coupled with a concern for their unique human needs. This is where ethics can help us get back on track.

Most of us make mistakes. If we're careful, we don't make too many, and our mistakes are usually correctable. But a legalistic obsession with avoiding or justifying mistakes will only increase the distance between ourselves and our patients. More useful than a detailed knowledge of the law is an experience of our patients as unique persons, with unique needs and unique values.

We'll be looking more specifically at the definition of ethics in the next chapter. For the moment, it's enough to say that ethics deals with our choices and actions toward others, looking for ways of expressing our deepest values through our actions. Avoiding litigation isn't one of the primary goals of ethics, but that may certainly be one of its side effects.

THE "BIG BUSINESS" OF HEALTH CARE

Health care has become a multi-billion-dollar industry. At the turn of the century, we spent very little on health care, chiefly because there was nothing to buy. Now we seem to have the opposite problem: too much to buy, too little to spend. The economic problems of health care are complex and interrelated. Depending on one's point of view, it seems that: no one is responsible, everyone is responsible, or everyone else is responsible.

Physicians, often unaware of the cost of the tests they order, or the size of hospital bills, feel little pressure to moderate their search for unlikely or untreatable diagnoses. Apparently unaware of the power of the pen, they may spend thousands of dollars (of other people's money) in a single day, oblivious to where that money is coming from.

Lawyers, pressured by an overcrowded profession, and riding a wave of generous awards in the courtroom, see opportunities for money to be made—the lion's share, of course, going to them. This in turn pushes physicians to order tests for legal rather than medical purposes.

Capitalizing on all this uncontrolled spending, corporations have sprung up to make money solely by offering "cost containment." These companies ostensibly make money by saving money, which is a nice idea. The so-called savings, though, frequently amount to something more like diversion. Are all these new companies saving us money, or just adding thousands of redundant jobs? Although it's a little early to tell, a healthy level of skepticism seems to be in order.

Health care for profit—there's money to be made out there. Unfortunately, the wages of the nurses seem to be "frozen," while the corporate salaries seem to be growing like proverbial weeds. The pressures of "unit value" freezes on physicians make them more introverted, more focused on their own expenses, more dissatisfied.

There's a bigger problem emerging here than just money. It's the distractions. We're distracted by seemingly pointless paperwork, by soaring costs, by the paranoid rush to "join up" with every new marketing idea so that we won't be "left out in the cold," by worrying about whether we will wind up in court because we didn't "cover ourselves" with tests. Pretty soon, we're exhausted and disgusted. Worse yet, there's hardly any attention left over for the patient, who's becoming even more disgusted than we are.

Is there a way out? When we cut costs, will all these problems vanish? Is there a magic HMO (Health Maintenance Organization), PPO (Preferred Provider Option), or corporate genius out there who can rescue us? Probably not. The real solution begins with recentering our attention where it really should have stayed in the first place—on our patients. If we really know our patients and their needs, spending their money with care comes naturally. If we know them as individuals, if there's a relationship of trust, we can forget about the courtroom.

Helping us to restore the relationship between ourselves and our patients is one of the benefits that ethics can offer.

THE QUEST FOR EXCELLENCE

Actually, our most pressing reason for studying ethics has little to do with the growth of technology or the pressures of the legal system. Most of us didn't pursue a nursing or medical education out of an intense love for hard science, or because we reveled at the thought of outwitting a hoard of lawyers. We started out with an embarrassingly simple emotion and the determination to carry it through. We said that we wanted to "help people."

In the process of memorizing chains of biochemical enzymes or the nuclei of the brain, perhaps we stopped voicing this humanistic ideal. But heaven help us if we stopped reminding ourselves of it. So the real reason for studying ethics is because we want to do the best we're capable of, making our original ideals more concrete.

Ethics can make us better at our chosen task of healing. Science can't tell us what to do when a patient asks to be allowed to die. Ethics doesn't tell us exactly what to do either, but it can point us in the right direction. It can help us pursue our involvement until we do find the best answer. Science doesn't know right from wrong. Ethics asks us to consider this question as an important part of what we do for a living.

Ethics can help us tackle difficult problems that we otherwise might have avoided or even failed to notice. It teaches us to be sensitive to the nontechnical aspects of healing. These topics receive only passing mention in our scientific education, yet they're centrally important to our daily work.

Ethics isn't just a public display of concern for right and wrong. It's a process of working toward consistently excellent choices. This process necessarily begins with the pursuit of inner maturity and personal growth. We might even go so far as to say that, for healing professionals, seeking personal maturity is an obligation, not an option.

Almost as a bonus, though, the effort we put into our professional growth can help us in our other personal activities. It can show us ways of improving the quality of our relationships with our families, our friends, and even our own selves. Once we become more aware of the meaning of our choices, we may recognize opportunities for growth that we would have missed.

Is all this just wishful thinking? No. Is it hard work? Yes. Does it require a tedious study of dusty philosophical texts? Not at all. What it requires is a recognition of our own personal resources for dealing with others, and a determination to use those resources to find the best answers to difficult problems.

In the process, ethics can help us enjoy what we do. It can make us more successful at the task of healing. It can restore our confidence in our own abilities. It can also restore our patients' confidence in the "system," and in us as its representatives.

Of course, ethics can't begin to work for us if we don't know what it's all about. Even if our intentions are correct, we can sometimes get lost among the practical details of a busy day's work. Recentering our attention can help. The next chapter will present a simple definition of ethics that we can return to when we seem to be losing our way.

It sometimes sounds as if ethics was recently invented, as if it were something new. In fact, excellent healers have always relied on ethics as a guide to their most important choices in dealing with others. It's a healthy sign that more and more nurses, physicians, and allied health workers are spending a little extra time trying to figure out what's best, even when the answers aren't easy or clear-cut.

Ethics isn't new, but recently we've become distracted by our marvelous tools, our own personal problems, and our hawklike (and often imaginary) adversaries. Yet personal concern and involvement have always been characteristics of the healing arts. The current interest in ethics demonstrates that the desire for quality hasn't been lost.

2   The Confusion about Ethics

Chapter 1 makes ethics sound positive, and it's certainly becoming a popular subject. But something doesn't quite fit. We've all heard or read about people whose experience of ethics has been less than enjoyable. Is there another side to ethics that isn't quite so positive?

For instance, some ethics committees we know of we'd just as soon avoid. In many states, a trip to the nursing or medical association's ethics committee can put us one short step away from being licenseless. In many hospitals, a complaint of misconduct brought before the ethics committee can make life truly miserable. In fact, it sometimes seems that, whenever someone else wants to give us advice, whenever they want to tell us what we *should* be doing, they call it ethics. Who needs that?

That kind of ethics sounds like an invitation for even more people to scrutinize our actions and second-guess our choices. It conjures up the specter of yet another "impartial" (meaning impersonal) committee designed to bedevil us with more rules; and when rules are on stage, punishment is usually waiting in the wings. Is there a dark side to ethics that we haven't looked at yet?

Actually, there isn't. But the word "ethics" has been greatly misused. If we're going to approach ethics properly, we at least need to have a clear idea of what it's all about. Once we have a hold on that, we'll be closer to seeing how much ethics has to offer us.

WHAT ETHICS IS NOT

Most of the confusion about ethics comes from the lack of precision with which the word is used. In fact, some of those who are most vocal about ethics would be hard pressed to define it. Before we look at what ethics is, we'd better spend a few minutes clearing the air. The following are topics for which ethics is frequently mistaken:

Rules of Business. When professionals become embroiled in an argument over money or business practices, one of the first epithets to surface is usually "unethical." This usage of the word really means, "I don't like what you're doing, but I guess it isn't illegal." This application of the word "ethics" is much too limited. It refers to arbitrary standards that can easily change. For example, ten years ago, a lawyer who advertised in the newspaper was considered to be acting "unethically." Today, advertising is an accepted practice within the legal profession. It would be more correct to call these rules "acceptable business practices," rather than ethics.

Codes of Performance. Every occupation, from real estate to television repair, seems to be devising "codes of ethics." Such written commitments to excellence show an admirable respect for quality. But having such a placard on our wall doesn't make us ethical—nor does adhering to its standards of quality. Being ethical isn't just a matter of performing a task correctly. Ethics is a much more internal, reflective activity. Certainly, ethics is interested in excellence, but not the kind of excellence that could ever be achieved by an efficient machine.

Enforcement of Local Rules. Sometimes the word "ethics" is used as a soft-sounding synonym for "reprimand." This type of ethics is usually one step removed from more severe punitive measures. Often mediated by unfriendly committees, this type of ethics is meant to strike fear into our hearts. If we pride ourselves on never having faced such an "ethics" committee, it's a sure bet that their actions really have little or nothing to do with ethics. Ethics isn't a tool for judging the actions or choices of others. In fact, the more sophisticated we become at ethical reasoning, the less judgmental we'll probably be. Ethics is much less interested in what others have done or are doing, than with what *I* can do to make my choices more meaningful and expressive of my most positive values.

Knowledge of the Law. There's a tendency for some of us to consider ourselves ethically informed if we're conversant with the latest Supreme Court rulings related to health care. Again, these are transitory standards that tend to reflect the present mood of society. Ethics is a more personal activity, one that can't be delegated to elected officials. The law gives us minimum standards for what is required or allowed. Yet, even if it's generally wise to act within the bounds of the law, doing so isn't necessarily enough. Ethics pushes us to go beyond minimums, asking "What is best?" In the end, the law is a part of the context in which we act, but it shouldn't be the sole determinant of our choices.

Adherence to Personal Principles. This is one of the most common (and dangerous) misconceptions about ethics. Many people, including many academic ethicists, think that being ethical simply involves voicing a set of moral principles and sticking to them, no matter what. This type of ethics seems to lean toward statements that begin with "I never . . . " or "I always. . . . " It's a serious mistake to think that we can ever really simplify our lives this way. The purpose of ethics isn't to devise rules that we can smilingly follow without a second thought. Its real aim is to give us the mental tools for living more creatively.

If we have set, unchanging answers to human problems, then we have a great deal to gain from our study of ethics. Although ethics urges us to think about what's best, it doesn't encourage us to face life armed with inflexible rules.

So why bother with rules or principles at all? Actually, in a more ideal world, there would be no reason. But most of us aren't capable of making all of our important choices from scratch, so we use rules as guides. However, when it appears that our rules aren't adequate to lead us to the best possible choice in a particular case, we should be willing to abandon them, or at least attempt to go beyond them. Those who never stray from their rules are like cooks who are unable to deviate from strict recipes. Their food may be edible, but it will rarely be memorable.

Also, devising rules can actually be good mental practice. It can help us refine our thinking and push us to identify our own preconceptions and inconsistencies. These are worthwhile activities if they contribute to a deepening involvement in life. But we still have to beware of letting the rules become the sole focus of our attention. Being able to mouth great ideals doesn't make us great persons (certainly a humbling thought to the authors).

Here is a brief summary of what ethics is not. Ethics isn't negative. Ethics is chiefly concerned with the pursuit of personal excellence, sometimes asking us to surpass ourselves. It encourages us to look for opportunities to learn and grow, rather than looking for pure safety.

Ethics isn't repetitive. It has very little interest in the mechanical application of rules. It has even less interest in forcing unique individuals to fit the mold of those predetermined rules. It thrives on creativity rather than uniformity. Ethics pushes us to be clever, finding choices that go beyond what we may have previously done or thought.

Ethics isn't just passive, wishful thinking: "If only things were a little different, I could do so much more." Instead of standing back, looking for excuses, it looks for ways of getting involved. Ethics isn't a spectator sport. All in all, ethics isn't just for ethicists.

Well, it's beginning to sound as if ethics "isn't this and it isn't that." Is it anything at all? Is there anything left? Obviously, the answer is "yes." The most important thing that ethics is not, though, is boring. Ethical reflection leads us to a deeper interest and involvement in life.

WHAT ETHICS IS

Ethics is a direct, focused interest in positive human values and their meaning, and an interest in making our values more real and effective through our choices. This sounds simple enough. Now are we finally ready to move on to the issues? Not quite. The problem is that we all tend to use common words without really understanding what they mean.

For example, the words "meaning" and "values" are ordinary enough—we've all used them without a second thought. Most of us, though, if asked to define them, would find it difficult to do more than give synonyms. Moving past this sort of mental complacency is what philosophy is about. It tries to get to the heart of simple concepts—and often it's the simplest ideas that turn out to have the greatest depth and richness of meaning.

MEANING AND VALUES: THE ROOTS OF ETHICS

In this section, we want to track our definition of ethics back to its most fundamental roots. After we do, we should have a clearer idea of where we're headed as we discuss our ethical ideas. We'll also be able to catch ourselves more quickly if we start heading down the path to "nonethics" again.

Meaning is a purely human invention. Animals don't need meaning in order to live. Animals simply live until they run out of the means to keep living. People are different. They *need* meaning in their lives. They need it just as surely as they need food or water or shelter. This is the most fundamental difference between people and animals.

The proof of this statement is simple. Animals never choose to stop living. Humans face this choice almost as a matter of routine. For most of us, the choice to stop living is rarely faced directly but it's always in the background. The choice isn't always dramatic, but it's always there.

Each of us is alive because we choose to be. Sometimes people choose not to continue living because they find no meaning in life. Occasionally, people choose to die because they find meaning in death. Animals don't make these choices. When they seem to choose death, they're acting only out of instinct or conditioning, not out of an awareness of meaning.

People need meaning. They may be comfortable and well-fed, but, without meaning, life is empty and flat. On the other hand, they can face almost impossible physical or emotional hardships, yet still find life rewarding and exciting—at least as long as they sense that their lives have meaning.

Meaning is what allows us to choose life over death (or death over life). *Values* are the *sources of meaning* in our lives. They are the concrete referents of human meaning. Human values are the specific focus of ethics.

People seem to be capable of valuing almost anything; they seem to be able to find meaning in all kinds of things and ideas. Consequently, we might jump to the conclusion that every person is always an ethical being—always trying to find meaning in his or her actions and choices. But ethics isn't just concerned with the existence of our values, but with their quality as well.

Not all values are positive and life-enhancing. Some values actually draw us away from ourselves and our inner human strengths. They weaken us and make us less capable. To be more correct, we should say that ethics focuses on human values that are positive. Ethics is interested in values which truly enhance our deeper selves.

It's tempting to try to draw up a catalog or menu of values, listing the "good" or "positive" ones in one column, and the "bad," "evil," or "negative" ones in another. Such a project, though, would be doomed from the start. Not only are people capable of valuing almost any thing or idea, they also seem able to value almost anything wrongly.

Here are a couple of examples. You and I both value money. You value it because of the freedom from worry that it gives you, and because having it allows you to do things that you believe are important. I, on the other hand, value money because it gives me a feeling that I'm important because I have it. I secretly look down on those who have less money than I do. For you, money is a positive value. For me, it is a limiting, negative value.

Of course, most of us realize that overvaluing material things can be dangerous—but what about "pure" values such as knowledge or truth? Aren't these things always good? Actually, these values can be the most liberating, but they can also be the most insidiously limiting.

Two academic mathematicians, known and respected, each place great value in knowledge. The first one, though, uses his books and ideas as a means of escaping the demands of the real world, eventually becoming more and more cut off from other people. The second, more alive, uses his mathematical ideas as a model to help him relate to the world and to other people. He seems to become more open and interested in life with each passing year.

The point is this: values don't really exist in the abstract, they always have a context. Their context is always a human one—the lives of real people. Values that lead us to choices that are limiting or immature are negative, weak values. Values that push us to grow in maturity and inner strength are positive. Ethics is really the science of positive, mature human values.

WHAT IT TAKES TO BE ETHICAL

Living an ethical life doesn't require special initials after our name. It doesn't demand a familiarity with important philosophical works. Being ethical doesn't even require that we use a certain specialized vocabulary.

What does it take to be ethical? More than anything else, it takes a desire to live a meaningful life, and an awareness that some choices are more meaningful than others. It takes a willingness to engage difficult questions, many of which don't have obvious or final answers.

If we're interested in pursuing meaning in our lives, how do we get started? What skills do we need? Most important is the ability to reflect privately in an open and honest way. We need to try to identify the most mature and lasting values we can. Then we need to look at the values that really motivate our daily decisions. Do our actual decisions demonstrate a firm hold on positive values?

As we grow more adept at self-reflection, we'll want to learn more about what others have thought. With their help, we can uncover inconsistencies in our own values and choices, and we can help them make progress, too. If we're open to new ideas, we can move much more quickly with others' help than we can alone. However, this attitude of openness needs to be tempered by a healthy skepticism. If we find ourselves or other people making important choices according to habit or convenience, we'll need to work to strengthen the foundation of those choices.

Holding and expressing positive values in a less than ideal world can be challenging. We want to succeed, not go down trying, so we'll need flexibility and an interest in trying new approaches. It takes creativity to live ethically in a practical world—a world that would be much more impersonal without our efforts.

Finally, living ethically will be easier if we have a sense of humor, a perspective about how much we can realistically expect from ourselves. Instead of seeing our failures as occasions to fix blame or find excuses, we should recognize our limitations for what they really are: markers of where we stand in the lifelong process of finding, of creating, meaning.

So, what does it take to be ethical? It takes a fair amount of honesty and hard reflective work. It takes a willingness to learn from ourselves and others, and an unwillingness to be fooled. As our talents improve, we'll learn to be more creative and flexible so that our values can be put to use in more and more difficult situations.

REFLECTION: THE FIRST STEP

Most of us have inherited worthwhile values from our families, our community, and our society. But these values aren't really our own until we've reflected on them and on their meaning for us as individuals. Even if we are "good" people, with good intentions, we won't really be "ethical" people until we've struggled to understand our values in the context of our own unique lives.

The process of ethics has two sides. Internally, ethics involves a reflective appreciation of our own personal values, always interested in making those values stronger and more meaningful. But ethics pushes us to get more involved in the public side of our lives, too. It encourages us to challenge our values by applying them to our everyday choices. The point is, ethics is concerned with living, not just thinking about living.

These two sides of ethics are equally important. Our inner reflection is like the training an athlete undertakes before entering into a public test of skill. The training is necessary, but it isn't enough. In many ways, it's the preparation that makes the challenge of public action even more compelling.

Personal reflection is the necessary preparation for ethical action. It makes us capable of ethical choices, but it also makes us want to get more involved as well. As Emmanuel Mounier observes, reflection is the ethical "diastole without which systole cannot occur."

Reflection isn't passive, it isn't a pulling back. It's an active and forceful effort to understand. Reflection looks at our experiences of ourselves and others and admits their importance. It looks at our successes and tries to find ways of repeating and generalizing them. It looks at our failures and tries to find ways of doing better.

Our personal system of values is the staging area for our important life choices. If the foundation is well-laid, our choices will be coherent and meaningful. If our values are merely inherited, or accepted because they sound good, our choices will be inconsistent, without real direction.

Since our lives don't stand still, our values don't either. Over the course of a lifetime, our values mature and grow. This doesn't mean that our youthful values are immature or wrong, but that they are the stepping-stones to deeper and more positive ways of facing life. If, year by year, our values grow stronger and more positive (not just louder), then the work of reflection is paying off.

For ethics, then, the world isn't just a stage on which events unfold. It's a milieu of human values, some positive, some negative. The purpose of ethics is to steer us toward positive, life-enhancing values that can hold lasting meaning for us. Part of the process of identifying and strengthening our values involves bringing them to bear on the choices we make each day.

Case 4

You recently took over the practice of a retiring pediatrician. One morning, a forty-six-year-old woman

brings in her fourteen-month-old daughter. The child
was born with a severe chromosomal abnormality, and,
in fact, wasn't expected to live this long. The child is
quite deformed, has little intellectual function, is severely
spastic, and is prone to recurrent aspiration pneumonias.
Her prognosis is bleak at best.

Today, the baby has a fever, is tachypneic, mildly cya-
notic, and has coarse noise in the right chest. You easily
diagnose pneumonia. You ask yourself, though, should
you treat it or not?

As a change of pace, let's discuss this case more thoroughly
before we go on. We already know enough about ethics to work
to a meaningful answer to this difficult situation. The facts are
fairly clear. This child has no real physical or psychological
future. Objectively, there isn't much to gain by treating the
infection. A deeper question remains: "Is there actually valid
personal meaning surrounding this small being's life—at least
enough to endure the pain and expense of medical treatment?"

This isn't a question that can be answered from a distance.
It could be that the mother is caring for the child only out of a
sense of hopeless duty, burden, and general frustration. Then
again, she may find satisfaction and meaning in demonstrating
publicly her love for her child. She may find subtle signs of
positive relationship in the touch of her child—or she may find
nothing at all.

The only way to find out more about what's going on behind
the scenes is to talk to the mother. The relationship we establish with her can give us the answers we need. Stock opinions
about severely defective children will only distract us from this
important resource.

It turns out that the mother, knowing that her child will
never live normally, still senses a bond. She recognizes signs
of awareness that the rest of us miss. She finds meaning in her
relationship with her child, and she has sensed meaning in her
daughter's life, too.

Still, she's becoming more and more convinced that the
meaning of her child's life is shrinking away, especially considering the suffering that the little girl must endure. She hates

the thought of losing her daughter, but she has an even deeper fear of the pain her child seems to live with. She surprises you by suggesting that the infection not be treated, so that her daughter can finally find peace and rest. You realize that withholding treatment can be a meaningful and positive action for you and the mother to make together.

The important lesson here is that we rarely make this type of difficult decision alone or in advance. In this case, the mother is as much a patient as the child; and the mother is our best resource for finding a positive, meaningful solution to a human problem that has many sides. The ethical work we do in this case won't tell us what to do in the next similar case, but it will help us improve our skills at getting the information we need.

When we lose sight of the goal of our actions, when ethics seems vague and unreal, we should return to the topic of human meaning. How can I act so that my actions bring meaning into my life? How can I help others find deeper meaning in their lives and choices?

SUMMARY

The greatest difference between people and other creatures is the human need for meaning in life. A life without meaning simply isn't worth living. The things or ideas that supply meaning to our lives are called values.

Each of us has a set of values that gives meaning to our lives and that guides our choices. No two people's values are exactly the same. Our values are affected by our upbringing, by our society, and by our experiences in life. Some of our values, even though they supply temporary meaning, weaken us and make us less capable in the long run. Other values are consistently positive. "Good" values are ones that enrich us as individuals and guide us toward inner maturity and strength.

Ethics is the conscious pursuit of positive values. It is based on honest reflection about our lives and our choices. Its purpose isn't to make life easy or comfortable, but to make it meaningful and worth living. It doesn't concern itself as much with what others should do, as with what I might do to find and deepen the meaning in my life and in the lives of those I'm around.

3 Ethics and the Health Sciences

So far, we've been discussing human values abstractly; now we need to be more specific. What are our deepest and most compelling values as healers? What meaning is there in what we do? Even though these are basic questions, they aren't necessarily easy ones to answer. In fact, most of us have a variety of values or goals that we bring to our work. On a practical level, we want to support ourselves and our families. That's a perfectly good value, but it doesn't distinguish health care from any other job. Yet we know, or at least we sense, that it *is* different.

On a deeper level, we may say that we want to "help those who are sick." Again, a perfectly worthwhile value, but just too vague. What does it mean to help people? What about the Boy Scout who "helps" the old lady across the street against her will? We need values that are simple enough to understand clearly, yet powerful enough to give our choices direction.

Having a firm grasp on our personal values can insure that we won't miss important opportunities for expressing them. It can help us get started again when we have "one of those days." It puts us a little more in charge of our lives, and it opens the door to discussing our values with others who've reflected as we have.

In this chapter we're going to give an example of some workable health care values. We say "example," because mature ethical values have to be developed individually by each of us; they can't be passively accepted from someone else. The ideas in this chapter do show, though, how this kind of work can be approached in a practical way.

ILLNESS VERSUS DISEASE

Before we proceed, a little background will help. There's a simple definition that has been useful to the authors in organizing their thinking. We'll be referring to this distinction frequently in the pages that follow: the difference between illness and disease.

Disease is a physical or psychological defect that can be described objectively. It can be known precisely (if our scientific tools are good enough), and its results are fairly predictable. *Illness* is the actual occurrence of disease in the life of a particular person; it's never abstract, and it hardly ever fits the textbook exactly.

As professionals, the majority of our training is spent studying diseases. We learn to recognize them through symptoms and tests, and we learn to treat them with proven therapies. Ideally, we all have access to the best, most current information, and we all make similar decisions. This approach is direct and it works. It works because diseases are more or less the same from one person's body to the next. But illness, the personal experience of disease, is very different from person to person.

Illness is an individual event—it's unique each time it occurs. Researchers deal primarily with diseases. Healing professionals deal with people who are ill. This difference is critical to understand, since dealing with an illness completely and excellently can require different skills than treating a disease.

The scientific model, so effective in battling bacteria, can let us down when our goal is to understand and work with complicated human problems—it trains us to confront problems armed with set strategies and recipe-like solutions. Yet the majority of difficult human problems can't really be understood from a distance.

If our attention is riveted on physical disease, we can find ourselves leaving quite a bit of our work unfinished. Of course, if we only want to be competent technicians and nothing more, then the scientific model is enough. But if our goal is to engage human problems at every level, we'll need a more inclusive model. Ethics asks us to be receptive to the bigger picture.

Case 5

Mrs. J is a thirty-two-year-old mother of two. She was in for her annual exam last week, and a routine cervical culture was sent. It returned positive for gonorrhea. You're surprised, but you tell her by phone that the problem is simple to take care of, and shouldn't do any lasting harm. You ask her to come to the office for treatment, and suggest that her husband do the same.

She comes in the following day, alone. You're a bit embarrassed and uncomfortable when she breaks into tears in your exam room.

Mrs. J has a fairly undramatic and eminently treatable disease. In fact, as diseases go, it isn't much. An injection or two, and it's gone. Her illness, though, may be more than she can handle. The sexual fidelity that has been an important value to her now seems a mockery. Her marriage, secure only a week before, is threatened by this previously unheard of bacterial culture. Even though her disease can be easily treated, her illness may be quite a challenge.

Disease affects only our bodies. Illness attacks us on many levels. Although illness usually begins physically, it often affects us psychologically or emotionally. It may threaten our self-esteem. Even after a disease has been treated or "ruled out," its threat may leave us less whole than we were before.

Even though illness affects us on many levels, it's hardly a unifying event. Through illness, our body can become our enemy. Illness can arrest our personal growth as individuals. It can distract us from our personal potential, making us more and more introverted, less and less capable.

Worse still, illness can reach beyond our physical bodies to injure those who are important to us. Illness doesn't seem to recognize the limits of the physical body. It spreads to affect families, friends, even those who are working to make us whole

again. Illness can breed anger and frustration, building a wall
around us. It can make us less attractive to others, breeding
resistance in all directions.

Luckily, like almost everything else, illness has another side,
the side that makes it a privilege to work with those who are
ill. Even patients who can't escape the destructive effects of
their diseases can be successful in dealing with their illnesses.
They can gain self-knowledge and self-confidence, finding inner
resources that even they never suspected were there. Being a
catalyst to personal growth can be a part of excellent health
care—a part that can be a reward in itself.

WHAT ARE THE GOALS OF HEALTH CARE?

A deeper question remains. What are we really trying to
accomplish? Are we just technicians staving off natural pro-
cesses, or are we something more? Could health care workers
someday be replaced by giant machines capable of fixing
diseased protoplasm?

Some still believe that the first purpose of health care is
simply to prolong human life. Most of us, though, realize
that this type of quantitative approach isn't enough. In fact,
some of the sorest criticisms of our health care system have
been leveled at its well-intentioned, but inappropriate, efforts
to prolong human life.

And so, another answer has become popular. We should try
to cure disease (when we can), and give comfort and support
when curing is impossible—"cure or care." Although these
goals are very reasonable, this kind of either/or thinking
eventually leads us down the road to professional, and ethical,
schizophrenia.

There are several problems with this model. For one, it's just
too difficult to know which task we should devote ourselves to.
Of course, we like to think that we can fully pursue both curing
and caring at the same time, but in practice our attention
usually goes one way or the other. Deciding to stop trying to
cure, when that's been our chief goal, can be soul-wrenching.

Another problem with "curing or caring" is the difficulty of
agreeing on the definition of curing. Can we really call it a cure

when important abilities must be sacrificed in order to continue living? One person's cure may be another person's curse. The word "cure" has a simple dictionary definition, but in practice it can be a very slippery term.

For example, consider the Jehovah's Witnesses who'd rather die than be "cured" by a blood transfusion. What we'd call a cure, they'd call assault and battery. Whose definition is right? Or what about the cancer patient who refuses the chemotherapy that offers a marginal chance for buying a few more months of life. Are they refusing a cure, or are we failing to offer one?

If we don't agree on the definition of curing, who should have the last word when important choices need to be made? Some believe that this responsibility belongs to the physician, who has both professional experience and scientific objectivity (some of you are wincing). Of course, anyone who has worked on the wards knows how much agreement there is among doctors about even the simplest of choices.

Trying to avoid these difficulties, some suggest that the goal of health care should simply be to do what the "consumer" says. Many times, though, patients don't want this honor, nor are they in any physical condition to make these major choices.

Case 6

Mrs. C is a sixty-eight year old nursing home resident, recently transferred to your hospital because of an upper GI (gastrointestinal) bleed. Her nursing home placement originally resulted from a stroke, which left her alert, but unable to communicate verbally. Conservative measures didn't stop the bleeding, so endoscopic sclerosis was tried. When that didn't work either, surgery seemed to be the only choice left. Mrs. C "communicated" with her facial expressions that she wanted everything done to save her life.

Surgery was performed, and the bleeding stopped. Unfortunately, it now seems impossible to wean Mrs. C from the ventilator. She has been in the ICU for two weeks, and there's no end in sight. She seems miserable. You're her

nurse, and you feel that something should be done to help
this poor lady, but you're not sure what.

Mrs. C's problems begin with the fact that we don't have the
right tools to cure her disease, but they certainly don't end
there. In fact, she now has a new problem: we can't seem to
decide what to do next. Focusing on either curing or caring
won't help her escape the predicament she's stumbled upon.
In order to succeed, we'll have to give up doing things "to" her
or "for" her and get involved with her unique individual needs
and values.

We can't cure everyone. So whom should we try to cure? Once
we've decided to try, how far should we go? These questions can
drag us around in circles, leaving us with a headache, but still
no definite answers. The rules of the game aren't at all clear. In
fact, they sometimes seem so slippery that they squeeze right
out of our hands just when we need them the most.

HEALING VERSUS CURING

One way around this confusion is to focus our attention a
little differently. There's a middle ground between curing and
caring, which really merges the two: *healing*. Healing simply
involves positive efforts to offset the damaging effects of illness.
This may sound like little more than a semantic distinction, but
it's a mental approach that can help us see all of our actions
as part of a unified effort. It's a mind-set that can cut our
confusion to a minimum. It encourages us to see all of our
positive actions as worthwhile and productive. The process
of healing is one of deepening involvement—it's *never* really
a pulling back.

Case 7

Mr. L is a lung cancer patient admitted with pneumonia. You're his social worker, but you don't see much good
in store for him. His tumor has encircled his aorta, and
it's invading his spine, causing him enormous pain. He's

already received palliative radiation, and chemotherapy seems to offer nothing.

Apparently denying his disease, Mr. L. still wants "everything possible" done to prolong his life, including "full code" status. The nurses on the oncology unit seem chagrined at the thought of doing CPR on this poor emaciated victim. You certainly agree with them, but you also respect Mr. L's right to make his own decisions. You find yourself praying that he will just slip quietly away in his sleep.

Our job obviously isn't to cure Mr. L—we don't have the means. It isn't necessarily to change him, either. What we need to do is try to understand him as he is, and help him do the best with the situation as it stands. He may not do as well as someone else, but, if we're excellent healers, he'll do the best he can.

The most destructive part of illness is the way it distorts our picture of ourselves. Illness can make our body our enemy. It can disrupt our relationships with others. Worst of all, it can threaten the sense of meaning in our lives. Uncovering and rebuilding this damage is the task of healing.

Healing is less limited than curing. It's open to curing, but never fixated on it.

· Even when nothing remains to be done for a failing body, the task of healing can still be wide open and inviting.

· Even when a patient's opinions are different from ours, there's still room for easing the effects of illness through a supportive relationship.

· Even when a dying patient is comatose and beyond our caring, the effects of illness can be dealt with as they affect family and friends.

· Even when there's no family, our healing efforts can be directed toward the other health care workers who've come to care about the patient.

· Even when death has finally arrived, the effects of illness often persist among the living, and the work of healing can continue there. Rarely, if ever, can nothing be done.

Healing isn't a complicated activity, although it's often a difficult one. It begins with our efforts to identify all of the effects of illness, and all of the resources at our disposal. The final, single goal is to make full use of those resources, so that our actions can be as effective as possible.

Healing doesn't focus on any single action or choice as the only right one. It inventories problems and resources and works toward countering one with the other. It remains success oriented, where curing can become focused on failure, setting goals in advance that are simply unattainable.

Once we've got a clear idea of what we're trying to accomplish, we'll find that we have fewer false starts, that we pursue fewer dead ends. Ethics can help. It directs our attention toward *meaning* as an important resource in the task of healing.

IDENTIFYING OUR PATIENTS

There are some practical implications here. If we're interested in human illness, instead of just physical disease, we don't need to confine ourselves to organs or even bodies. We can look deeper for opportunities for healing. Moreover, since disease can damage the lives of all who contact it, we can still find opportunities for healing even when there's nothing we can do for a failing body.

Also, the person whose body is diseased may not be the only one who's ill. At times, family members may be as much our patients as the person whose name is on the front of the chart. Sometimes health care workers (including ourselves) will become patients because of our involvement with a person who's ill. It's perfectly appropriate to pursue our healing role with all these people. In fact, it's inappropriate to ignore them.

Case 8

You're the on-call physician in a major hospital Emergency Room. You're called to attend to Mr. D, a seventy-one-year-old gentleman transferred from a rural facility.

The story you receive is that he underwent a lower limb amputation a few days before. Postoperatively, a period of severe hypotension apparently caused infarction of a segment of small bowel. The referring doctors hope that hyperalimentation might help him, and that he might even recover—that is, if their diagnosis is wrong.

At the present time, Mr. D is "out of it." He doesn't seem to know where he is, and he doesn't seem to know what's happening to him. His wife aggressively demands that "everything be done" for her husband, including major surgery. Two surgical consultants, whom you respect, concur that surgery might well be lethal. His wife, though, presses you to find "someone" who'll do the surgery. The nursing staff is beginning to choose up sides.

In this case, and a great many others, the disease begins in one body, but now affects several other people. Mr. D's disease is a problem for his wife, which she can't seem to cope with. In fact, the situation is taxing the physician's resources, and, before things work themselves out, it may affect many others as well. Perhaps family members will appear who disagree with what's being done. Like Mrs. D, they may be "ill" because of Mr. D's disease. The hospital staff members are already finding themselves drawn more and more deeply into the problem.

The point is this: even if we can't find much to do for Mr. D, we may be able to do quite a bit for the others involved; and that's an important part of our work. We may be able to help his wife adjust to this sad situation (which would certainly be an achievement). Or we may be able to help each other deal with our frustrations and feelings of inadequacy—bringing something worthwhile out of a situation that on the surface seems purely negative.

Applying our values in difficult situations is what ethics is about. Finding ways to express our values can be difficult, but with cleverness it can be done. These aren't scientific skills, learned in a laboratory, but human skills that we learn together. They're the result of an interest in making our personal values visible in an otherwise impersonal world.

WHAT ETHICS CAN OFFER

Ethics is more like a map than a shortcut. It helps us see more clearly where we are and where we want to go. It can even suggest ways of getting there; but it can't guarantee that the path will be easy.

Ethics is the science of meaning. Its orientation is toward finding meaning in life through our inner reflection, and toward expressing our interest in meaning through our choices. Its goal is to lead us toward mature personal values that can have lasting meaning.

Health care ethics, as a practical branch of ethics, is a joint venture in finding and expressing meaning. It focuses directly on the needs of patients, but its raw materials are the personal values of all those involved. What makes this process so challenging is the fact that the answers that work for one person may not work for another.

People who are ill have very specific, practical needs. They often face situations and choices that are new to them but that simply can't be avoided. Because health care ethics is practical, it isn't interested in abstract theory which sounds good but doesn't work. When ethics is performing the way it should, it leads to better decisions, ones that express the most positive human values available to us.

Even though ethics won't help us be better scientists, it can help us be better healers. It can teach us to recognize human problems more quickly so they can be dealt with more effectively. It can help us identify the inner strengths of our patients, so these strengths can be used when they're needed. It can help us locate our own personal resources and use them more predictably.

Ethics can keep us interested in excellence, and help us avoid being suffocated by our failures. It can help us learn to measure our actions against realistic expectations, protecting us from perfectionistic demands. It can help us find ways of accomplishing a great deal, even when science fails to give us the means to cure.

Because health care ethics is interested in unique answers, it can be a creative activity. It can give us the opportunity and skills to put the cookbook aside, participating in ethical decisions that occur only because *we* are there. Although others might arrive at similar results, the ethical process always bears the creative stamp of the unique individuals who have worked together to solve a shared problem.

THE ETHICAL APPROACH

In Chapters 6 and 7, we'll outline some of the ethical theories that have been proposed for dealing with ethical dilemmas. A philosophical model can help organize our approach to problems, but it can't do the work for us. Regardless of which "system" we choose (or even if we reject them all), there are certain practical steps which are important to our success.

Defining Our Own Values

At the risk of being repetitive, this critical step can't be overemphasized. We don't inherit strong, positive values. We find them through private reflection, and we strengthen them by putting them on the line in our day-to–day activities. Inner reflection is a life-long commitment for those who hope to live ethically.

Recognizing the Opportunities

Another important step in the ethical process simply involves recognizing when a problem exists. Although this may sound too basic to bother discussing, it can actually be one of the most useful skills we can develop. Training ourselves to watch for the subtle red flags that go up when things aren't going the way they should can get us off the sidelines and into the game.

Some of the red flags are obvious. When three different people are telling us that we "must" do different things at the same time, it isn't hard to see that trouble's brewing. Or, when our own personal needs or values seem to run directly counter to another's, a showdown is probably coming.

These occasions can be either nuisances or opportunities. "I need an abortion," can be bluntly dismissed by, "I don't do them." The same statement, though, can be recognized as an invitation to help with a difficult personal choice. Sometimes, even though we can't do what people want, we can still help them with their deeper personal needs.

Even more subtle, and difficult, are the situations where we recognize a problem before it has broken out into public view. Death, the consummate unknown, is one of the most common red flags for the healing professional. The proximity of death can often be felt by health care personnel long before it's apparent to laypersons. This knowledge can be used to help identify and strengthen personal resources before the last minute.

Chronic illness, a constant reminder of our mortality, often has the same impact as the threat of death, yet it's frequently underestimated. Staying alert to some of these less dramatic warnings of a coming problem can allow us to get personally involved sooner than we otherwise would.

Following Through

Telling others what we think is right or wrong isn't really what ethics is about. "Being there" for the whole journey is. In fact, carrying our decisions through can sometimes be more important than the decisions themselves.

When things seem to be going sour, our strongest impulse may be to stand back, to insulate ourselves. Ethics encourages us to get even more deeply involved. Practicing our ethical and reflective skills, we can sometimes help patients use their limited time to work more quickly and surely toward a meaningful answer.

The next four chapters present a condensed version of the philosophical underpinnings of biomedical ethics. It should be clear by now that learning to use a certain vocabulary doesn't make us ethical. Even though the authors certainly have their own bias, there's no approach that is categorically right or wrong. The final purpose of studying theory isn't to help us "choose up sides," but to stimulate our own thinking, to push us ahead.

4   The Vocabulary

When people specialize, narrowing their area of interest, inevitably a new dialect sprouts up. Health care ethics is no exception. Fortunately, there aren't many new words to learn—but if we're constantly hearing them without knowing what they mean, we can feel left out or intimidated. Of course, peppering our speech with three- and four-syllable words doesn't begin to make us ethical. But using words correctly can facilitate our dialogue with one another. It can make our exchange of ideas more efficient and less prone to misunderstanding.

For simplicity, we've divided this vocabulary into three categories: principles, terms, and issues. Ethical principles are philosophical concepts that can be used to analyze problems. "Terminology" includes some everyday words that take on special meaning in ethical discussions. Issues are topics of controversy and are discussed in the next chapter.

The dividing line between these groups isn't always clearcut. For example, the principle of autonomy is fairly simple: it refers to our individual right to make our own choices. Most of us would agree that this is a worthwhile idea. But let's say that Mrs. Smith wants an abortion, and Dr. James believes that abortion is morally wrong. Both of them may cite the principle of autonomy in his or her own behalf. The principle of autonomy now becomes an issue. The fact that these two people agree "in principle" doesn't save them from the pain of grappling with their conflict of values.

THE PRINCIPLES OF ETHICS

These days, it's rare to attend a forum on health care ethics without hearing at least some mention of ethical principles. Usually, the principles being referred to are those of Kantianism: autonomy, beneficence, and justice. A more complete description of Kant's ethical theory can be found in Chapter 6.

Autonomy: The Right to Choose, the Right to Refuse

Coming from root words that roughly translate into "choosing for ourselves," this idea asserts each individual's right to set his or her own moral course in life. It urges us to allow others to make important choices for themselves, instead of trying to decide for them.

For example, let's say we're discussing treatment alternatives with a patient. The patient surprises us by opting for no treatment at all—a choice that we ourselves wouldn't make. The principle of autonomy encourages us to support that choice in spite of our disagreement.

Saying that someone's decision is "autonomous" has a positive ring. Everything else being equal, it's usually a good idea to let others make their own choices. Unfortunately, an autonomous choice can still be morally wrong, so supporting someone's autonomy doesn't excuse us from examining the quality of their decisions.

When we say a choice is autonomous, then, we aren't really making a judgment about correctness or appropriateness. A decision can be considered autonomous if we make it on our own, regardless of whether others consider it right or wrong, and regardless of the good or bad results that choice finally produces.

Beneficence: Doing Well

Health care is a practical activity—results are extremely important. Beneficence refers to an inner motivation toward accomplishing positive results through our actions. One way of appreciating this word's meaning is to contrast it to the related word "benevolence." Benevolence simply refers to "meaning well," regardless of what finally happens. Beneficence goes a big step further. It asks us to direct our choices so that we achieve results that are "good" or "right." It suggests that having good intentions simply isn't enough in the ethical arena.

The concrete effects of this principle are subtle: we should act so that we truly envision a good or positive outcome to our actions. If we accept this orientation, we lose the security of being able to excuse our failures by pointing to our noble motives.

Justice: Equal Treatment for All

The Principle of Justice encourages us to treat everyone alike. It asks us to be consistent. Instead of trying to solve important human problems on the fly, justice pushes us to develop rational solutions which we can use over and over. Again, this principle doesn't tell us what to do, it only tells us how to go about it. In fact, we can act very wrongly, yet still be quite "just."

For example, let's say we decide that everyone over the age of sixty-five should be "put to sleep," to make room for the next generation. If we apply this rule consistently (including getting into the extermination line ourselves), we are being just. Obviously, we are also being "just" plain wrong.

A word of caution. The imposing ring of the word "principle" can fool us into thinking that our decisions are better simply because we've referred to them. These principles, though, are really just tools for analyzing our problems; they rarely, if ever, provide us with clear-cut answers. Certainly, they can be useful, but if they narrow our thinking too much, we're probably better off without them. And so, if someone says, "You're clearly violating the Principle of Justice," our first impulse may be to apologize and promise to do better in the future. A better reaction might be to ask ourselves, "So what?"

THE TERMINOLOGY

The following terms frequently come up in discussions of health care ethics. They have specific meanings that might not be obvious if we're hearing them for the first time.

Cost/Benefit Ratios (Risk Analysis): Tipping the Scales

Trying to discuss theoretical "principles" with a patient can sometimes confuse matters without gaining much ground. Instead of being abstract, we may choose to analyze our alternatives in a very practical way, looking matter-of-factly at the pluses and minuses.

Almost every medical procedure has a good side and a bad side. For example, let's say that Mr. Jones has metastatic cancer of the colon. Radiation and chemotherapy don't have much to offer. Surgery isn't likely to cure him either, but at least it will probably provide some physical relief. For Mr. Jones, the immediate question is whether the pain, expense, and risk of surgery are worth the benefits that they offer.

When we start trying to weigh the good news against the bad news, we're doing risk analysis. Although this has a scientific sound, often the "factors" involved are fairly subjective. The pain of surgery may not be a major problem for Mr. Jones, but for someone else it may be very forbidding.

On a social level, this kind of homework can be very useful. Risk analysis can help us decide where best to spend our time and money. Like the actuarial work done by insurance companies, cost/benefit ratios can be used to apportion our limited resources in the most appropriate and productive way possible.

Paternalism: The "Big Brother" Mentality

The antithesis of autonomy and free choice is paternalism. This refers to the tendency of some of us to believe that we're uniquely qualified to make important decisions *for* others. In most cases, the target of this criticism is a physician, but other professionals, or even family members, are sometimes fingered.

Examples of paternalism include the withholding of critical information from a patient because he or she "wouldn't be able to handle it," or telling a patient what he or she "should" do without presenting alternatives. In general, paternalism suggests a condescending attitude.

The Living Will: Choosing Ahead of Time

A living will is a written contract between a patient and his or her health care providers. Its purpose is to help direct that patient's care in the event that he or she loses the ability to communicate. For example, Mrs. Parker signs a living will stating that, should she be rendered irreversibly comatose, she doesn't want to be kept alive by artificial means. Later, after a massive stroke, Dr. Brown uses the living will as legal and ethical support for his decision to "pull the plug."

A living will can be very specific. It can say that intravenous feedings are acceptable, but that mechanical ventilation isn't. Or a living will can be quite general, simply stating that "unreasonable" means to prolong life shouldn't be used. The specific wording of a living will is left up to the patient and his or her physician—but the intent is the same: to protect both of them in the event that critical decisions have to be made without the patient's input.

Competence: Licensed to Choose

"Competence" refers to the *capacity* to choose in a mature fashion. The fact that we have this capacity, though, doesn't necessarily imply that our choices are mature, or good, or correct. It simply means that we're capable of appreciating the major effects of our choices.

Similarly, saying that someone is legally "incompetent" isn't an insult, but simply a description. The legally incompetent individual is one who can't appreciate the importance of the choices he or she makes. For example, a person with advanced

Alzheimer's disease might be declared incompetent due to his or her impaired memory, even though that individual may be quite functional otherwise.

The really difficult problems come up when we aren't sure whether someone is competent. The person with mild mental retardation who refuses surgery is a good example. Even though their choice might seem reasonable to us, we still have to wonder if they really understand the impact of their decision. If our doubts are strong enough, we sometimes find ourselves turning to the courts for a final determination.

Informed Consent: The Right to Know

Consent forms have become a familiar sight in hospitals and clinics. They provide written evidence that procedures have been explained to patients, and that they've freely chosen to undergo them. Even though consent forms are simple documents, the idea of free and informed consent is fairly demanding. Having a signed consent form in the chart doesn't necessarily prove that informed consent has been obtained. Several conditions generally must be met:

1. Our description of the procedure should be understandable; technical language should be avoided.
2. A reasonable description of the benefits of the procedure should be offered, balanced by a description of common discomforts and hazards. The amount of detail contained in this disclosure usually relates more to the urgency of the procedure than to its risk. For example, an elective procedure, such as cosmetic surgery, may require more extensive disclosure than a truly life-saving, yet more dangerous surgery.
3. A description of alternative treatments, including nontreatment, should be given, along with their potential benefits and risks.
4. Coercion should be avoided. Examples of coercion might include statements like "If you don't have this operation, I can't be your doctor anymore," or "If you don't let me do this for you, you'll certainly die."
5. There should be an effort to solicit questions, and to determine that the patient indeed understands the information that has been

presented. (Polite nods and a signature don't necessarily prove that someone even speaks English.)

The Harvard Criteria: Re-defining Death

For generations, the medical definition of death centered around the automatic function of the heart. With the advent of high-tech emergency care, especially CPR, this definition quickly became obsolete. In fact, the heart is commonly turned off and on in the course of cardiac surgery.

In 1968 a team of neurologists at Harvard University re-defined the medical concept of death, basing it solely on neurological function. The so-called Harvard Criteria requires that there be an absence of coordinated activity by neurologic examination, as well as a flat line on the electroencephalogram (usually done twice at a twenty-four-hour interval). Medical factors that could obscure the clinical picture, such as drug overdose, must be ruled out.

This new criteria of death, though, has already come under fire. The Harvard Criteria requires that there be both loss of higher cortical function, and loss of brain stem activity (e.g., spontaneous respiration and pupillary responses), for the diagnosis of clinical death to be made. But is spontaneous respiration or a few waves on an EEG sufficient to constitute human life? Many ethicists are currently looking for an even better way of defining human death.

Institutional Review Boards (IRBs): Unseen Watchdogs

Public and private hospitals are the testing ground for much of our medical research. In fact, clinical trials are usually required before any new drug or procedure is approved for general use. Monitoring the safety of these human experiments is the job of the IRB.

Most of our large hospitals have IRBs, but their work isn't often made public. These committees include a balance of laypersons and health professionals, each member bringing a slightly different perspective and background to the group.

IRBs evaluate research proposals to determine that they're well planned and organized. They review the consent forms used in research projects, to insure that they're understandable and complete. They monitor the results of ongoing projects, to guarantee that they're safe.

The powers of the IRB are extensive. If it refuses to allow a research project, or demands that one be terminated, there is often no recourse. Even if a project is fully funded and ready to proceed, the IRB must be satisfied that the study is well-organized and potentially beneficial to its participants. If the IRB isn't convinced, the clinical trial may be over before it begins.

Ordinary versus Extraordinary Means

The words "ordinary" and "extraordinary" are common enough, but they have different meanings to different people. To nurses and doctors, extraordinary treatments are investigational or unusual ones. In ethical circles, the term "extraordinary" tends to mean "unreasonable" or "excessive." This inconsistency can lead to quite a bit of confusion.

For example, Mr. Gatti is only forty-four years old, but he has an unusual chest cancer that has resisted complete diagnosis and treatment. The outlook is bleak. When respiratory failure occurs, Dr. Kaplan calls for the ventilator. Medically, that might be considered an ordinary treatment. Ethically, it's extraordinary, since there seems to be so little to gain.

Also, the boundary between ordinary and extraordinary doesn't stand still. Fifteen years ago, kidney transplants were clearly "extraordinary"; today they're almost routine. If we plan to use these terms at all, we'll probably want to qualify their meaning.

Whistle-blowing: Speaking Up

Nurse Jenkins is frustrated by Dr. Becker's unprofessional behavior. He's slow to answer his pages, and difficult to deal with when he finally calls. He sometimes leaves town on weekends without arranging proper backup. Finally, she goes to the hospital administration with her complaints. She's "blowing the whistle," exposing Dr. Becker's failings to an authority above him.

Whistle-blowing goes beyond back-room gossip. In most cases it involves a subordinate formally criticizing his or her superior to a higher authority. Sometimes it even involves exposing problems to the news media or to legal scrutiny, especially when normal disciplinary channels seem to be ineffective.

Blowing the whistle isn't to be taken lightly. Since the target of the complaint usually is in a position of authority over the whistle-blower, some sort of "negative feedback" is to be expected.

These are a few of the words that frequently come up in ethical discussions. In the next chapter, we'll look at some of the issues that provide grist for the mill of ethical debate.

5   The Problems and Issues

"Ah, they're finally getting to the meat." Unfortunately, discussions about ethical issues are more like a menu than a meal. They can whet our appetite for getting more involved, but they rarely satisfy our hunger for answers.

In this chapter we'll be cataloging some of our ethical questions. In fact, by the time we're finished, it may seem as if there are just too many questions to even begin finding answers. Yet meaningful answers can certainly be found. In Chapters 6 and 7, we'll look at some of the ethical systems that have been used to work toward them.

The issues in this chapter can be argued from at least two points of view—that's what makes them issues. Consequently, if we choose up sides, we're bound to find ourselves standing opposite some good, logical arguments. But if we're continually appreciating everyone else's opinions, we may find ourselves trapped into immobility.

Indecisiveness isn't what ethics is about. These questions have to be answered—maybe not in final or absolute ways, but at least in practical ways that help us do more for those who face these problems in their everyday lives.

Public debate can be very productive. It can help us inventory our questions. It can expose us to the insights of others, keeping us alert to the complexity of these sensitive topics. Yet, in the long run, the real aim of ethical debate isn't to win, but to learn.

EUTHANASIA: THE RIGHT TO DIE

Euthanasia literally means "good death." It comes in two strengths: active and passive. Active euthanasia involves intervention that is specifically intended to hasten death. An example would be the use of a general anesthetic to bring a terminal condition to its conclusion.

In the Netherlands, for example, it isn't uncommon for people with terminal illnesses to choose death by means of a lethal injection, bypassing the weakness and suffering of their last days. To say that this form of euthanasia is controversial is an understatement. In fact, when we witness a truly heated debate about euthanasia, it's almost certainly about the active form.

Passive euthanasia is more commonly called the withdrawal of medical support. An obvious example would be the decision to turn off the ventilator that sustains a comatose person. Also related to passive euthanasia is "nonintervention" (e.g., the decision to let a final pneumonia take its course). Passive euthanasia has been an accepted practice for generations. Active euthanasia hasn't.

Is there really a difference between writing an order to discontinue IVs and writing an order to deliver a huge dose of a potent narcotic, especially when we know that the final outcome will be the same, except for a few days of lingering? Some say that we're only fooling ourselves when we allow the withdrawal of support but deny treatments that could prevent days or weeks of agony.

Proponents of active euthanasia point to its compassionate motivation, and to its ultimately positive results. They decry the injustice of withholding this type of relief from those who find no religious or philosophical value in prolonged suffering. They argue that the simple availability of this type of treatment can make many individuals' final days more tolerable, even though few will actually make use of it.

To opponents of "good death," though, there's nothing good about it. They see it as a first step in a dangerous and morally destructive direction. To them, active euthanasia changes the whole character of the healer's role in society. It opens the

door to the scientific pursuit of death, instead of the focused
pursuit of life.

Moreover, they point out, once this first step is taken, it won't be long before physicians and nurses will be taking these matters into their own hands, "choosing" death for those who might not make that choice on their own. The long-term result of the active pursuit of death will inevitably be a deterioration of the moral fabric of our society, or so they suggest.

At the heart of this issue is the principle of autonomy. Should competent adults be allowed to choose treatments they see as beneficial, even if others might disagree? Some of the staunchest advocates of patients' rights still find themselves drawing the line short of active euthanasia. But do our misgivings about this issue really make sense, or are they just holdovers of a simpler era?

ABORTION: WHOSE RIGHTS COME FIRST?

The abortion controversy has been smoldering for decades. The polar positions are well known: "right to life" versus "pro-choice." But the hidden issues are complex, defying easy answers. Unfortunately, this problem stubbornly refuses to go away.

The debate centers around the ambiguity of fetal life. When does the fetus become a person? Some say at conception. Others say only after the vital organs have formed (around the sixteenth week of gestation). Some maintain that viability (usually after twenty-four weeks) is the beginning of personhood. Others say that birth (at whatever gestational age) is the true beginning of a person's life.

What criteria should we use to settle this disagreement? Some argue their position by referring to religious beliefs, some turn to the legal system, and some look for scientific answers. It's almost as if each side is speaking a different language, and there are no translators to be found—everyone's got something to say, but there's no common ground.

When does the embryo or fetus deserve the minimal right of protection from harm? Answering this perennial question would provide at least a little momentum toward a positive and consistent approach to abortion. As things stand, we seem to be angrily pushing against a brick wall in the dark. Is this an unanswerable question, or are there already *too many* answers?

Even if we could decide who the players are, we'd still have to decide which positions we're going to let them play. Does society have the *same* duty to protect the unborn life that it has toward the child who's already been born? Or are there different levels of protection owed to different people?

For example, what about the commonly accepted "therapeutic" abortion of children with birth defects, such as Down's syndrome? Is a person with such a condition automatically less than a person, and therefore outside of the state's protective eye? Are there levels of personhood even among viable fetuses? Indeed, some consider it malpractice *not* to offer abortion to a mother carrying a child with Down's syndrome. If so, should we also allow parents who accidentally bear Down's babies the option of putting them to death? How far should we let logic carry us?

There are purely practical arguments to consider as well. We live in a real world; abortions *will* be done, regardless of our opinions. Is it morally right to place our theories above the safety of these women? If we return abortions to the back room, are we simply sacrificing a different group of lives?

We can't begin to solve this problem until we agree on some basic definitions. When does human life really begin? Is a human fetus the property of its mother, or is it only in protective custody? When there's a conflict of needs between the mother and the fetus, whose responsibility is it to weigh the merits of those needs? Until we can agree on answers to these questions, the problem of abortion will continue to divide us.

CONFIDENTIALITY: WHO HAS A RIGHT TO KNOW?

Case 9

Mr. K, a homosexual, has been admitted for a relatively routine surgery. His surgeon has a policy of sending a screening test for AIDS, on all high-risk patients. As his nurse, you're afraid that the result of the test will be posted in his chart, and will be seen by people who have no right to the information.

You decide to tell Mr. K that the test's been ordered. He says that he doesn't really care, as long as no one tells him the news. You're surprised, but you decide to respect his wishes. Unfortunately, the test comes back positive. Now you wonder about your responsibility to Mr. K's present and future sexual partners. Do *they* have a right to know? Do you have an obligation to tell *him* in order to protect *them*? If his sexual partner appears on the scene, should he be told, against Mr. K's wishes?

The confidentiality of medical information has a long and proud history, but how far should our respect for this ideal carry us? Do we sometimes have an obligation to reveal information to people who could be hurt by *not* having knowledge that we possess?

Examples of this type of dilemma are becoming more and more common. For example, a patient who carries a serious genetic disorder doesn't want anyone to know about it, even though this information might be crucial to relatives who could also be affected. Do they have a right to know? The fiancée of a patient with a serious psychiatric illness knows nothing about his history. Should we tell her?

Another growing problem of confidentiality concerns our private medical records. Many hospitals have fine print in their admission forms that allows researchers to screen charts at random for data collection. How confident are we that the information they find won't leak? Many insurance companies keep computerized records of patients' diagnoses. Do they really have a right to that information?

Some argue that our private medical records are an extension of ourselves, and therefore shouldn't be allowed into the hands of people who aren't in a position to help us directly. Others say that medical information is a social resource, and may be used freely. In the middle, most of us don't care much, as long as our medical records aren't used against us. But should we care a little more?

TRUTH TELLING

Mrs. Fisher has cancer. Her family says that she'll "just give up" if she finds out. Is it perhaps better for her not to know? Can't knowledge of the truth sometimes be destructive? Then again, if we hold back, are we demeaning her dignity and taking away an opportunity for growth?

Carrying this question a little further, what about the patient (like Mr. K above) who "doesn't want to know?" If we decide that it isn't fair to withhold information, do we have to go the next step and *require* that patients be told the truth against their protests?

How much detail is required to satisfy our notion of telling the truth? For instance, a patient asks, "How many months do I have left?" Knowing that our answers are unreliable, should we still quote statistics, or is it alright to evade the question? Just how specific do our answers have to be in order to be considered truthful?

But the issue of truth-telling goes even deeper. When we witness professional misconduct, should we convey that information to the patient, or is it alright just to ignore the problem? When *we* make a mistake, should we volunteer to discuss it, or is it acceptable to wait (fearfully) for patients to find out on their own?

And what about the tricks of the trade? What about the bland statement that "This won't hurt (much)," or the common practice of introducing medical students as "doctors"? What about the tradition of giving placebos to patients without their knowledge—are these just sanctioned forms of lying?

Do we have to tell the truth, the whole truth, no matter what? Or is it ethical to mislead people a bit if we're convinced that knowing the truth isn't really in their best interests? More and more people are moving away from the "caring lie," but is the alternative always better?

CONFLICTS OF RESPONSIBILITY: THE LIMITS OF LOYALTY

From the outside, the health care team often appears to be a smoothly functioning, well-coordinated unit. Behind the scenes, though, it's as human as any other group. Most of the time, differences of opinion don't detract from the quality of patient care—in fact, they often improve it. But what should we do when we firmly believe that bad decisions are being made?

For example, you're a night nurse on a busy medical-surgical floor. One of your patients is having a rough night, and you fear that he won't live until morning unless something is done soon. Unfortunately, the patient's physician doesn't seem interested enough to come in from home. Should you respect his professional role, or press the issue?

Some say that the "team" can't function without an identified and respected leader, presumably the physician. They say that internal conflict only weakens the ability of the group to function. In the end, this hurts the patient more than anyone else.

Others say that respect must be earned. When someone is wrong, they are wrong, and social roles can't change that. If the nurse is a professional, then there's a time and a place for independent thinking, for taking a firm stand. That time and place comes when the patient is receiving less than adequate care.

Carrying this question a little further, what should we do when we sense a serious conflict between the dictates of the law and the needs of our patients? Most of us shy away from the thought of a direct confrontation with the legal system, but is there a time to consider a public showdown?

As an example, consider the controversy over the right of nursing staff members to strike for improved working conditions or higher pay. Some argue that the continuity of hospital care is too important to jeopardize for the sake of political issues. Others point out that, when conditions are poor, it's the patient who suffers the most. Either way we go, it seems, we're wrong.

We feel ourselves pulled in different directions. Sometimes our various loyalties and responsibilities threaten to pull us apart. When do we stand up for our deepest beliefs, and when do we just roll with the punches?

RESOURCE ALLOCATION: THE COMPROMISES WE MAKE

How can we spend our limited health care dollars in the most efficient way possible, and still be fair? This is the issue of resource allocation. Although often considered a topic for debate, this problem is really just a fact of life, and it's a question that confronts us on many levels.

On a limited scale, consider what happens when two critical patients arrive at a rural hospital at the same time. The staff knows that they can't handle both cases at once. Should they do the best they can for both patients, probably losing them both? Or should they concentrate on one, and let the other one go? If they decide to save only one, whom will it be? The one who has a little better chance of surviving? The one who arrived thirty seconds earlier? The one who has the bigger family? Or the one who's more likely to pay the bill?

Although this is a small scenario, the same drama is enacted on many larger stages. For example, an HMO is deciding which services it will make available, and which will be left out. Should kidney transplants be offered at the expense of educational programs to stop smoking? Should screening mammography be allowed, even if it means that immunizations will have to be cut?

We can't do everything for everyone—we have to make compromises. In the case of that HMO, should the decisions be made according to what the consuming public seems to want? If so, diabetic education might lose out to sports medicine. Or should we decide what's best for everyone, and offer that regardless of marketability? If so, our enrollment figures may not allow us to do much for anyone.

On an even broader social level, should we allow research money to pour into heart transplants, when we haven't brought health care for the poor up to par? Then again, do we need to balance our efforts on all fronts in order to succeed?

The issue of resource allocation frequently returns us to an age-old question. Is health care a right or a privilege? If it's a right, *how much* of it are we entitled to as individuals?

TRANSPLANTATION ETHICS

We're rapidly moving into an era where the transplantation of vital organs is medically routine. This has created some exciting new possibilities, but it has also raised some difficult new questions.

Since transplantable organs are a scarce commodity, how do we decide who will get the benefit of their use? What safeguards should there be to protect the prime donor from having his or her organs "harvested" a bit too hastily? What about the big business of brokering organs for money: is this a life-saving enterprise, or just another disgusting scam?

The following case is hypothetical, but it's bound to come up. Mr. Braun is a healthy forty-seven-year-old man. His sixteen-year-old son is slowly dying of an incurable cardiomyopathy. A heart transplant is the son's only hope, but an unusual blood type makes this seem unlikely. Mr. Braun has no other family, and has "no desire to go on living in a world without his son." He wishes to be the donor. Will we let Mr. Braun make this sacrifice for his son, or will we deny him even a hearing? If we don't anticipate some of these new problems, we may find ourselves with just too little time to deal with them when they do come up.

DEFECTIVES: HOW FAR SHOULD WE GO?

A child born with a severe mental or physical handicap, who probably won't survive without extraordinary treatment, is a "defective." Obvious examples are the infant with meningomyelocoele (spina bifida) or hydrocephalus. Although we have treatments for these problems, our treatments still yield very mixed results.

Sometimes our therapies lead to almost miraculous cures. Other times they only prolong and magnify the physical suffering that nature might limit by an early and merciful death.

In between lie the majority of cases, where we gain a little, but at enormous human and economic expense.

Unfortunately, we can't always predict which child will profit from our treatments, and which one will only suffer from our intervention. When we withhold treatment, we can't escape the haunting fear that we may be sacrificing a salvageable, meaningful human life. Yet if we give in to this fear, and treat "all comers," we still have to face the additional physical and financial misfortune we've created.

How do we strike a balance between our reluctance to sacrifice a single human life, and our reluctance to prolong the suffering of those who really have nothing to gain? How can we learn to face these decisions day-in and day-out without becoming emotionally drained or hardened?

GENETIC ENGINEERING

We're moving more rapidly toward Aldous Huxley's "Brave New World" than even he could have imagined. We already have the technological skills to analyze much of the genetic information in the nucleus of the human cell, and to insert modified DNA into specific locations. This is the topic of the President's Commission Report, *Splicing Life*.

Using these new techniques, we can identify the genes responsible for the transmission of genetic diseases and correct them before fertilization occurs, insuring that these diseases won't be passed on to future generations. Although we might not be able to undo the damage done to those already born with these disorders, we'll be able to guarantee that their children won't be affected. The potential is staggering, but the risks are awesome as well. Our biggest question at this point isn't "Can we?" but "Should we?"

Proponents of this research say that the gene pool (the genetic material of the breeding population) is a social resource, and that society has an obligation to future generations to protect it. They say that we've already done too much to contaminate the gene pool by keeping those with serious genetic disorders alive until their childbearing years. Now we have a responsibility to clean up.

Their opponents say that this type of technology is just too dangerous for the human race to handle at this point in history. They liken genetic engineering to the advent of the nuclear age. Although there is the potential for accomplishing much that is positive and beneficial, in the end genetic engineering will probably be turned toward more selfish and destructive ends.

They say that this scientific revolution will really be the most dangerous Pandora's Box ever opened. In creating the raw materials for our project (human-infective viral particles), we will also be inventing the ultimate in germ warfare. Even if our intentions remain pure, we can't avoid the risk of accidentally unleashing viral plagues that could destroy or change the human race as we know it.

They also say that genetic engineering is the first step toward a socially destructive master-race mentality. We'll ultimately lose our respect for individuality, for nature, and for God—becoming arrogantly uniform, as we change the human race to fit our own short-sighted image of what we think we ought to be.

Actually, this debate may be irrelevant. Throughout history, we've developed new technologies as rapidly as we could, regardless of the risks, and genetic engineering isn't likely to be the first exception. How can we control this compelling, yet terrifying, new science? How can we keep from becoming our own worst enemies?

THE ENDLESS MARCH

The above issues are important and pressing, but there are still dozens we haven't mentioned:

· Is surrogate parenting a way of providing excellent homes for children who would otherwise never be born, or is it just a subtle form of buying and selling human life?

· Is it ethical to conduct clinical experiments on prison inmates, military personnel, or patients in mental hospitals? Are they coerced by their circumstances into participation?

· In fact, is it even ethical to experiment on laboratory animals, especially when the research has questionable value?

· Involuntary sterilization: is breeding an inviolable human right, or a privilege based on a certain degree of personal responsibility?

· The DRGs (Diagnostic Related Groups) and other governmental regulations: how much should we allow them to affect the care that we give?

· Is the free market, where the pursuit of profit sometimes outweighs humanitarian ideals, the proper place for the development of new drugs and techniques?

Even if we could learn to ignore these issues, they won't go away. We can't tackle each new problem with a clean slate, without exhausting ourselves early in the process. What we need are ways of unifying our approach to these issues so that we can set a positive and consistent course for our future. That's why we turn to ethical "systems," which are the topic of the next two chapters.

6 Five Traditional Approaches

Even if we've only started to identify the ethical questions facing us, it's natural to want answers. "Ethicists," we tell ourselves, "spend years discussing these problems. They must have solved them all by now." Sad to say, that's not so. In fact, ethicists can be just as perplexed by these issues as the rest of us, but they have an edge. They have logical, methodical approaches, and that's what we want to investigate in this chapter.

In the next few pages, we'll be looking at several accepted and commonly used philosophical approaches to ethical issues. No one of them is clearly accepted as the most worthwhile. Still, each can be useful if it helps us see problems we would have otherwise overlooked. Unfortunately, each of them can also become a mental trap if it stops us from reflecting further about our ethical problems.

For the sake of example, we'll "test drive" five common ethical approaches on the following everyday case. Of course, a single case is hardly an adequate test for an entire system, but a trial run can give us a feeling for how these ethical theories perform in practice.

Case 10

Mr. R is seventy-eight years old, and a prominent man in the community. Tonight, on the way to a speaking engagement, he was involved in an automobile accident that resulted in a closed head injury. He is comatose, on a ventilator, but his pulse and blood pressure are strong and steady.

The neurosurgeon, consulted to attend to Mr. R, says that immediate surgery has less than a 10 percent chance of returning him to a state of reasonable function. Also, a living will, only a few months old, appears prominently at the front of Mr. R's clinic chart.

The family, though, is in disagreement about what to do. The eldest daughter says that her father wouldn't want to live in a handicapped state, and that he should be allowed to die in peace. The wife says that the living will doesn't apply to this situation, because it happened so suddenly. The rest of the family is quiet, but very concerned.

This case raises some interesting questions. The right-to-die issue is conspicuous, but we'll find it difficult to verify Mr. R's present wishes. What was he really thinking when he wrote his living will? There are several individuals strongly affected by Mr. R's accident, but some of them seem unwilling or unable to make their thoughts public. Do they know something we should know? Let's see if ethical theory can help us.

DEONTOLOGY: OUR DUTIES TO ONE ANOTHER

The word "deontology" comes from the Greek word *deon*, meaning duty. This approach should appeal to those of us who appreciate logical structure. It sees ethics as a set of rules that can be followed in the same way by all of us, all of the time.

The historical roots of this system trace back to the writings of Immanuel Kant in the late 1800s. Kant believed that the rules of ethical behavior are built-in to the human mind, but that it takes work to learn to use them. Helping us to understand these innate rules better is the job of ethics.

As deontologists, our task is to uncover ethical principles that are good, organize them logically, and carry them through consistently. When we're finished, we should have a system that can be followed by any "good" person, without a lot of hesitation or rethinking.

For Kant, our ethical duties come in two forms. Absolute (or perfect) duties are ones that apply to all situations. To him, the clearest example of absolute duty was his famous Categorical Imperative. The title of this rule is a little intimidating, but the concept itself isn't difficult. Kant's highest law says that we should always make those choices we would want others to make. Kant put it this way: "I ought never to act except in such a way that I can also will that my maxim should become a universal law." (Direct statements weren't Kant's strongest suit.)

Since this idea is so close to the biblical notion of "Do unto others . . . ," Kant's Imperative is sometimes called his Golden Rule. In fact, almost every culture in history has, at one time or another, voiced this ethical principle— perhaps proving that certain ethical rules are truly inborn.

Modern deontology isn't too strict about following Kant's terminology, even though his method is respected. Therefore, Kant's Categorical Imperative has been subdivided, expressing the same idea in a more manageable way. The Principle of Autonomy tells us to respect the rights of others (just as we would want them to respect ours). The Principle of Beneficence tells us to act so that our choices achieve truly good results. And the Principle of Justice urges us to treat everyone in a similar manner.

These rules are more or less universal. We should be able to follow them all of the time, regardless of the circumstances. So far, so good. But now the hard part. Some ethical principles are not quite so universally applicable. These involve relative (or imperfect) duties.

Examples of relative duties are easy to come by. For instance, keeping our promises is ethically important (the Principle of Fidelity), but it isn't hard to think of situations in which we "should" break a promise. Let's say we witness an accident while on our way to a birthday party. Even though we've promised to go to the party, we "should" stop to lend a hand, even if it means that we'll have to break our earlier promise.

Or take the general rule which states that we "should" tell the truth (the Principle of Veracity). Sometimes we still have to think twice before acting on this rule. For example, a Nazi SS squad appears at our door asking if there are any Jews in the house. Given the situation, it might be wrong (unethical) to tell the truth, even though honesty is usually right.

This is where the deontologist really earns his or her keep. It's one thing simply to list the rules of ethical behavior, but quite another to structure them in such a way that they lead us in the right direction all of the time. Obviously, a huge heap of rules won't do, and changing our priorities as we go isn't acceptable either.

For example, we might agree that it's wrong to steal. But would it be morally right to steal a loaf of bread in order to save a helpless child's life? Most of us would accept that—placing the principle of respect for human life above our respect for property. But would it be morally right to steal the starving child, in order to provide a better home for it? Some of us might balk at that. When is stealing to protect human life alright? How can we organize our rules so that the same order applies to every case? Priorities are the real key to deontology.

In this approach, then, the ethicist is very important. He or she organizes ethical rules so that the rest of us can make more sense of them. In a way, the ethicist is only telling us what we already know (since the rules are built in), but the knowledge is now arranged so that it's clearer, and can be used more confidently.

In effect, deontology asks us to do the difficult work of ethics ahead of time. It says that the human mind comes with ethical principles of behavior as standard equipment. The goal of formal ethics is to organize this knowledge so that it can be understood and applied consistently by everyone.

Going back to the case of Mr. R, we'll want to find a way of dealing with his problem that would apply to *every* similar situation. The Principle of Autonomy, focusing on his living will, would seem to push us toward letting him die. Of course, we'll still have to figure out what to do about the autonomy of his wife, the nurses and doctors, and the other members of the family.

The Principle of Beneficence seems a little easier to satisfy. It asks us to achieve a good result. However, some of us might argue that death is never good, even when living is difficult. We may need some other principles to reinforce our feeling that death can sometimes be a positive value.

The Principle of Justice tells us to treat Mr. R the same way we'd treat someone else who isn't as prominent or influential. The fact that his wife might threaten us with legal action shouldn't sway us if we're really committed to doing the right thing.

For the deontologist, the case of Mr. R isn't exactly easy, but it's manageable. However, we may find other deontologists who agree with us in theory, yet disagree with our conclusions—a situation that could be an embarrassment to the system. In the end, we'll probably let Mr. R die peacefully, since that seems to show the most respect for his rights as a mature individual.

CONTRACT THEORY: LET'S MAKE A DEAL

This approach is really a variation of deontology, but one that minimizes some of its drawbacks. Contract theory says that we should follow predetermined ethical rules, but that they don't have to be innate to be correct. The rules of ethics are what we agree they are, pure and simple. This ethical system mirrors John Rawls' social theories. It has a flavor much like that of our Western legal system, making it easy for most of us to relate to. With contract theory, we agree to agree about our ethical rules, then we stick to them no matter what.

Where Kant asks us to search the recesses of our ethical minds to discover inborn rules, contract theory says that the rules of ethics are a product of consensus. By living in society with each other, we automatically accept the power of the group to make rules that apply to us all. Interacting with each other, we implicitly accept mutual limits on our behavior.

But how do we avoid accidentally making (and following) bad rules or agreements? We do best by standing back, taking a rational, disinterested point of view. We eliminate our self-interest—or at least we try to. We act fairly, and with impartiality. Justice is very important to contract theory.

On a social level, contract theory is fairly clear-cut. Our society has certain rules. If we choose to live here, we must follow those rules. But in our individual dealings with each other, contract theory can be a little ambiguous. Are we expected to put every move, every possible outcome, into writing? Obviously this won't work. Instead, we pay attention to the implicit contract that occurs whenever we deal with others.

In the case of health care, for instance, patients have certain reasonable expectations of their providers. The providers also have expectations about what their patients should do. The sum of these expectations provides the basis for an implied contract of performance. In practice, this works fairly well until problems arise.

Unfortunately, when things aren't going just right, contract theory has a double disadvantage. On the one hand, both parties have already adopted a legalistic, rigid mind-set. This predisposes to conflict. On the other hand, the implicit contract is usually too vague to provide much structure. This leads to confusion and misunderstanding.

In the case of Mr. R, though, contract theory makes our decision quite easy. We've agreed with Mr. R ahead of time about what we should do in a situation like this one. Now we just do it. If others protest, we have an earlier, rational agreement to refer back to. Done.

UTILITARIANISM: WEIGHING OUR CHOICES

What if we'd rather avoid the work of defining moral principles altogether? If so, utilitarianism is for us. This system presents a balance-sheet approach to ethics—it should interest those of us who enjoy mathematics.

Utilitarianism is concerned solely with the *results* of our choices, not our motives. As a "result," this system happily avoids the headache of establishing moral definitions of right and wrong. In utilitarianism, right is what works. As an added bonus, this approach requires far less philosophical background than the others.

In any given situation, there are usually several choices we could make. Different choices lead to different results. As utilitarians, we try to foresee these results as well as we can, then make the choices that lead to the greatest overall happiness (or the least unhappiness) for everyone involved.

For example, let's say that we've decided to divert our funds for indigent health care into small business loans. Utilitarianism doesn't have any problem with that, as long as it can be shown that such a move results in a greater total amount of human happiness. With utilitarianism, we don't really have to deal with abstract questions of right and wrong, good and evil. We just concern ourselves with consequences. Utilitarianism basically says that doing the right thing for the wrong reason is perfectly okay. What really matters is what we accomplish, not our fine intentions.

However, utilitarianism isn't totally free-wheeling. In most utilitarian systems, we're still expected to decide ahead of time which results we consider to be most productive. The difference, though, is that we don't have to justify our choices by pointing to consistent moral principles. We justify them solely by the sum total of human happiness we achieve.

Again, we try to be as objective as possible. When we ourselves fall on hard times, we shouldn't try to overemphasize our own needs. As utilitarians, we strive for impartiality. This means considering our own happiness to be equally important to everyone else's, but not more important.

The key to being a good utilitarian is proficiency at recognizing all of our options, and accuracy in foreseeing the probable results of those choices. If we're good at predicting human behavior, we should be successful utilitarians.

The biggest advantage of utilitarianism over deontology is its flexibility. Sometimes we sense that a certain decision is best, even though we can't quite explain why. As utilitarians, we won't have to search for abstract reasons to explain our choices. We can just point to our (excellent) results.

The biggest disadvantage of this approach, though, is that it allows quite a bit of room for rationalizing bad choices. "Well, I just thought that (such and such) was more important in this case than (such and such)." In the end, it's just too difficult to quantify and compare human values and needs. Focusing entirely on our own priorities can actually lead to unpredictable, and sometimes arbitrary, results.

In the case of Mr. R, our first job as utilitarians is to list all of our possible choices, and predict what would happen in each case. For instance, if we let Mr. R die, his wife might take us to court—certainly causing a dip on our own happiness scale. This is what utilitarianism might euphemistically call a "disvalue."

If we operate on Mr. R and he does well, we'll have achieved an excellent result. Unfortunately, the odds are against us. However, if we operate, and he does poorly, he may suffer a good deal. But at least his wife will be satisfied; and we ourselves will be out of danger—that is, unless one of the quieter family members decides to go after us for not honoring the living will.

So what will we do? Perhaps we'll find ourselves recalling Marc Antony's famous lines from Shakespeare's *Julius Caesar*: "O, that a man might know the end of this day's business 'ere it comes. . . . "

SITUATIONALISM: LOVE WILL FIND A WAY

Situationalism, based on the reflections of Josef Fletcher, was popular in the 1960s. Fletcher proposed that choices made out of unbiased love for others are good choices. In this system, the unselfish act is the highest type of ethical behavior.

Situation ethics is so named because it sees each ethical situation as being truly unique. It says that moral principles and laws that try to fit every situation only approximate what's really best. If we want to produce really excellent results, we have to tailor our solutions to fit individual cases.

Fletcher's approach is said to be modeled after the teachings of the New Testament. It is often (and probably wrongly) seen as a variation of utilitarianism. Like utilitarianism, situation ethics says that we sometimes need to modify our ethical choices to fit the particulars of a given case. However, situationalism is far less cold and abstract. To Fletcher, it makes no sense to call ourselves "good" simply because we follow rules or laws correctly—even if those laws are basically good. We should call ourselves good only if we consistently act out of love for others.

As situationalists, we won't willingly sacrifice the welfare of an individual for the sake of upholding a moral or legal rule. When our loving intentions dictate a choice that conflicts with the law, it's the law that must bend.

For example, let's say that our job involves destroying food surpluses from government warehouses. A passerby in need catches our attention, and we listen to her story. Although our action is technically illegal, we still decide to help out, instead of quoting our duty to uphold the law. Even so, this one decision doesn't mean that we have to do the same for everyone else who walks by.

In this model, we use our ethical choices to express our most loving intentions toward others. Here, ethics is the clear teacher and master of the legal system, and we don't allow rules to stand in the way of making the very best, most human decisions we're capable of.

Of course, we still have to be careful to distinguish the *real* needs of individuals from their *perceived* needs. Sometimes we all want things that aren't really best for us. In situation ethics, we aren't always bound to do what people want—we do what's best for them because we love them.

The most common argument against situationalism is that it allows us to justify almost any kind of behavior on the basis of a private emotion. It's just too easy to believe that we're acting out of love, when in fact we're acting out of habit or unrecognized self-interest. This is a system that is somewhat lacking in objective limits.

Going back to Mr. R once again, there's really only one critical question for the situationalist: "What's the best (most loving) action to be taken in Mr. R's behalf?" Operating or not operating isn't really as important as the *manner* in which we carry out our choice. In fact, whatever we decide to do will be right, if it's done lovingly.

VIRTUE THEORY: THE ANCIENT APPROACH

Virtue theory should be enticing to those of us who are enthusiastic about self-help. The most famous advocate of virtue ethics was Aristotle, as handed down to us in his *Nicomachean Ethics*.

In an ethics of virtue, we focus our attention on our own personal character. Our ethical ambition is to develop inwardly, to grow in virtue, so that, in the end, we're "as good as we can be." As followers of Aristotle, our first task is to reflect on the meaning of "strength of character." What personal qualities are most important to us in our quest to be "good?" Simply listing these qualities isn't enough, though. We have to understand how they work together.

Personal character is really a blend or mixture of opposites. Take consistency, for example. Although it's generally good to be consistent, we can carry this virtue to excess, becoming compulsive and myopic. Consistency needs to be balanced by flexibility. Having too much of one trait can turn a virtue into a vice.

In other words, true strength of character involves finding a middle ground between complementary elements—balancing one quality with another. This is implied in the ancient dictum of "all things in moderation." Nearly any personal characteristic can be a virtue (if balanced), or a vice (if unbalanced).

After we've thought about the human qualities that are most admirable, we need to begin developing them. In a way, this sort of ethics is like weight lifting. By methodically developing our skills, we'll eventually be able to do more and more.

An ethics of virtue is really an ethics of habit. Choices are opportunities for developing good habits. By pursuing excellence in even the most routine of situations, we'll be prepared for more difficult problems. The choices we want to make, then, are the ones that will move us most surely down the path toward inner strength. In this sort of system, choices that strengthen us as individuals, that help us grow and mature, are good choices. If we are good, the ethical decisions we make are, almost by definition, good.

If we want to deal with Mr. R's problem in a virtuous way, we'll do what a "good" person would do—whether anyone else likes it or not. In the end, our dealings with Mr. R and his family will probably be very positive for us. This case gives us opportunities for balancing bluntness with tact, compassion with firmness, hope with realism, and so on. In the end, we're likely to profit greatly from our contact with these unfortunate people. What finally happens to Mr. R isn't all that important anyway, is it?

CONCLUSION

Actually, the above ethical examples are just a sampling of the ethical theories available to us. There are several others, but they've attracted less attention than the ones sketched above. Because our descriptions have been brief, there's a short bibliography at the book's end to guide further reading.

There's one common ethical pitfall we should warn against: namely, the practice of using different approaches in different situations. After just a little practice, it isn't hard to figure out where each system shines. Succumbing to temptation, we can find ourselves changing theories like clothes. This is called ethical eclecticism, and it essentially puts us right back where we started.

We come to ethics for answers. If we have to compensate for the weaknesses of one ethical theory by substituting another one in a pinch, we should question whether we've gained anything at all. In fact, when we recognize that it's time to change theories, we're really just demonstrating that we can do better on our own.

In the following chapter, we'll introduce an approach that we believe has much to offer. It's tailored to fit the needs of healers more than theorists.

7　The Personalist Approach

We've all met excellent healers, people who somehow seem to know just what to do in difficult situations. What's their secret? Are they really the most logical deontologists, or the most efficient utilitarians? Even more to the point, each of us has achieved excellent results ourselves—but maybe we're not so sure how we did it. Were we following one of the systems in the last chapter without knowing it, or were we just lucky?

Which of those approaches really captures the essence of ethics at its best? Actually, all of them have one problem in common, a flaw so fundamental that it can't be overcome. They all draw our attention away from the people we're dealing with, focusing us instead on abstract ideas.

Kantianism and contract theory direct us toward preconceived rules, utilitarianism toward specific results, situationalism toward our own feelings, and virtue theory toward our personal character. In the end, they all fail because they distract us from something that is even more important: the needs and values of the people we're dealing with.

Personalism, based on the writings of several modern French philosophers, is different. It doesn't ask us to be coldly rational about our responsibilities to others; it encourages us to get involved on a personal level. It also says that some of our choices are better than others, that there are right and wrong answers to our problems.

Personalism is an ethics of relationships, not rules. It says that human problems can't be excellently solved using inflexible principles or logic. People aren't machines, and they don't respond well to being treated as if they were. Personalism asks us to find creative answers to unique human problems. Our best resource here isn't cold logic, but our own ability to approach other people as individuals.

THE DEEPEST HUMAN VALUE: RELATIONSHIP

In Chapter 2, we said that meaning is what ethics is all about. We admitted that people sometimes find meaning in all sorts of things and ideas, but we also suggested that some sources of meaning, some values, are more mature and worthwhile than others. Our best approach to ethics should be based on an understanding of the most solid and lasting of human values. But what really makes life meaningful? At times, we all make the mistake of thinking that what we own is what matters. Most of us eventually realize, though, that possessions don't really satisfy our innermost needs.

Some of us, a bit more cerebral by nature, slip into a similar mistake: thinking that ideas or opinions are the most meaningful part of life. Of course, ideas can be stimulating, and sometimes they really do add to our lives—especially when they help us know ourselves and others better. But ideas aren't (or shouldn't be) the deepest source of meaning we can find in life.

There's something very simple and basic that is more valuable than any possession or idea. Our most positive and lasting meaning comes from the quality of our relationships, with ourselves and with other people. The proof of this statement can be found in our answer to the following simple question: on our deathbed, looking back, will we find that life was worth living because of what we've owned or thought, or because of the people we've known and the quality of our relationships with them? A personalist ethics succeeds or fails according to how we answer this question. If we believe that personal relationships are the most meaningful experience in life, we're personalists. If we try to explore this idea, to organize our thinking, then we're being philosophical about the subject.

AN OVERVIEW

The fundamental guide in this type of ethics is a deep respect for the importance and worth of each person we meet. In working with others, it isn't the problem that's most important, and it isn't a set of abstract principles that counts—it's the people who matter most.

When an ethical red flag goes up, a personalist ethics doesn't turn away to reexamine lists of logical rules or principles. It turns directly toward the people involved, to try to better understand their personal values and their individual needs. To measure the quality of our ethical decisions, this approach looks at how well our choices demonstrate respect for all those involved, including ourselves. Often, the best measure of this respect is the depth and quality of our involvement.

Dealing with other people in an honest way requires an acceptance of their uniqueness as individuals. Even when we don't agree with what we find, we can't make progress until we accept what's there. Our most powerful resource in approaching others isn't cold logic or impartiality, but our ability to relate to people as individuals—to understand their needs, values, and potential in a personal way.

In order to become constructively involved with the values of others, we have to be in touch with our own. This means reflecting deeply and honestly about what we think is really meaningful in life. Our goal is to weed out values that are superficial or weak, replacing them with values that are consistent with our belief that people are more important than things. Then, when we think that our values are solidly understood, we'll want to put them to work. Even our simplest dealings with others provide opportunities for demonstrating our respect for them. In fact, what we do in ordinary situations can be more revealing than how we handle a crisis. When people bother us over small problems, when they don't seem to understand, when they are nuisances, our ethics is put to its severest test.

In our daily routine, a personalist ethics keeps us focused on quality, rather than just getting by. It helps us recognize problems earlier, so they can be dealt with sooner and more effectively. It encourages us to take seriously problems that others might consider trivial or unimportant. It also reminds us to be available even after our technical job is finished. But this ethical approach also excels in difficult or unusual situations. People seldom make critical life choices according to the rules of logic. Therefore, when a special problem arises, a personalist ethics doesn't ask "What rule do I need?" but "Whom do I need to know better in order to understand what's best to do?"

To answer this question excellently, we need to use our own deeper abilities. The ones we need most are interpersonal skills: listening, understanding, and communicating effectively. We want to be able to get involved, not just stand at the sidelines giving advice.

Using our personal talents, we can learn more about those who are caught up in a crisis, and with persistence we can appreciate their problems as if they were our own. In fact, as we enter into a relationship of trust with others, their problems really do become ours.

Is this too dangerous an approach? Will taking on others' problems eventually overwhelm us, grinding away at our energies until we're exhausted? Not if we openly accept their help as we go. Drawing on their strengths, and contributing our own, problems can be solved much more reliably and successfully than if we try to do the job alone.

Personalism isn't difficult to learn, but it can be challenging to apply. The best personalist is the one whose day-to-day activities show an unswerving respect for people. This demands, above all, a recognition of each individual's uniqueness and special worth. A personalist, then, is basically an expert at achieving strong and open relationships with others. This isn't a talent that is learned overnight, but it can be learned. It is a creative ethics, one that never seems to runs out of surprises. Receptive to the values of others, our own values are constantly challenged and refined. Engaging the problems of others, we find and develop personal resources which would otherwise be less complete.

THE THEORY

It may sound as if personalism is just a general attitude. Is there a theory here too? Actually, there is—a rich and inviting one. Personalism studies our everyday experience of relationship, and gives us ways of improving our skills. It also gives us a vocabulary that helps us exchange ideas and insights more effectively.

This isn't a theory that dwells on telling us exactly what to do. Instead, it looks at what's already going on, and helps us find ways of doing even better. In this theory, two words constantly come up: person and relationship. These are everyday words—ones that most of us use with hardly a second thought—but once we start looking at them a little more closely, we'll see that they're far from ordinary. As we learn more, we'll also see that our knowledge can be put to good use.

Knowing what a person really is, we won't find it quite so agonizing to decide when to turn off the ventilator—and we won't be so likely to turn it off too soon, either. The same definition can make it easier to decide which defective infant should be allowed to die peacefully, and which one should be given everything we've got. Also, knowing what goes into a strong and workable personal relationship, we'll find the approach to others more accessible. When we don't know what our responsibilities are, we'll have a way of getting the information we need—namely, by coming to know the people we're dealing with.

Person

We all know that a person isn't just a thing, like a car or a brick, but what does it really take to be a person? A certain physical appearance? A minimum IQ? A few organized waves on an EEG? An immortal soul? It's amazing how little agreement there is about this "simple" definition. Actually, there are three abilities that are unique to people, which things and animals don't have: a conscious self, personal freedom, and personal promise. Reflecting on the meaning of these capacities can help us understand and appreciate what it means to be a person.

The Self. The unseen relationship of self-awareness isn't just a poetic notion, it's the central experience of being a person. The self is a constant dialogue that permeates all of our experience. Although we consciously direct this energy at times, we never control it completely. Even when this dialogue is broken (during dreamless sleep or anesthesia), its potential is still there. When the potential is lost, so are we.

Case 11

Mrs. T is one of your favorite patients. She's a delightful seventy-seven-year old lady who's had only minor medical problems in the past. On the morning of admission, she was found slumped in her chair at home, apparently the victim of a massive stroke. Her deteriorating condition caused her to be placed on mechanical ventilation in the emergency room.

Now three days have gone by, and she's off the ventilator, but there's still no sign of improvement, except for her spontaneous respirations. You're sad to see her in such a state—you wish you had a living will to help guide your decisions.

The potential for self-awareness is the *sine qua non* of personhood. In the case of Mrs. T, is there a realistic chance that she will regain her inner relationship with herself, her self-awareness? Even though we might not be able to answer this question at the beginning of her illness, each passing day gives us more information. Yesterday's decisions don't have to back us into a corner if we're willing to face this important question again and again.

The answers to some of our most difficult ethical quandaries hinge on our definition of the human person. Even though we don't have the scientific tools to measure self-awareness exactly, we almost always have a sense of its presence. When this crucial capacity has been permanently lost, our physical efforts can still demonstrate our respect for that person's memory, but the time for life-or-death decisions is past.

Freedom. Another fundamental difference between people and animals is the existence of human freedom. Although this definition is hotly debated by philosophers and scientists, few could seriously deny that human freedom exists. The strongest proof goes back to a fact we mentioned earlier—namely, that people sometimes choose to stop living, a choice animals really can't make. The positive side of human freedom is even more important: people live because they choose to. Although we aren't always aware that we are choosing to live, we have to admit that we *could* choose to stop living. For humans, life itself is an act of choice.

However, our personal freedom pushes us far beyond just choosing to live or die. People bring their freedom to bear on nearly every facet of their experience of life. The deepest, and most important, side of freedom has to do with choosing values and relationships that have meaning for us, and taking a stand there.

The patient who's come up against an untreatable terminal illness may seem to be out of choices. In fact, though, such an illness can be an occasion for a person's most profound expression of human freedom. In other words, our freedom isn't necessarily defined by the number of choices we have, but by what we do with the choices we've got.

Promise. The third crucial element of personhood is personal promise. Each of us, no matter how simple or sophisticated, has the capacity for inner growth, for changing in ways that lead toward inner maturity and personal strength. Most of us easily recognize this quality in children, but too often we lose sight of it in ourselves and other adults. Yet, as we grow into adulthood, so does our promise.

Personal promise is more than just a bland admission that there's always room for improvement. It's an actual part of us, as real as our memories or imagination. Moreover, fulfilling our personal promise isn't just a vague possibility, it's an individual need. Of course, this need can be ignored, but that won't make it go away. Coming to accept our potential, and our limits, we come closer to understanding who we are as individuals.

The following simple case illustrates all three of these elements of personhood.

Case 12

Mr. and Mrs. S are surprised and horrified that their newborn daughter has Down's syndrome. The child is fairly severely affected by her trisomy, and you don't envy these parents' situation. When they are told that the child also has a relatively minor heart defect that requires surgery, they seem almost relieved. "It's God's will that this baby die," they tell you. "If God wanted her to live, He would have given her a normal heart."

The most critical question here points us back to the definition of the human self. Is this baby potentially capable of self-awareness, of sharing in meaningful relationships inwardly and with others? Is there a realistic chance for this baby to find meaning in life? Most likely, our answer will be "Yes." If so, Baby S is fully a person, not just a mistake of nature.

Our problem, then, may center more around the parents than the child. What's influencing their reaction to this unexpected event? Are there other children in the family whom they think will suffer from having a retarded child in the home? Are there worries over the expense of heart surgery, problems they're reluctant to discuss because they might sound too cold and uncaring?

Actually, there's a deeper problem here, one that hinges on human freedom. The parents, anxious to avoid making a decision about this difficult problem, would rather place the responsibility on God. In so doing, they're missing the fact that the problem indeed belongs to them. They do have choices, and their best choice will be their most meaningful one. God hasn't decided for them. In their efforts to avoid the problem, they may be missing an important opportunity for personal growth and maturity. Helping them explore their own resources, helping them accept responsibility, may be our greatest contribution to this difficult situation.

Relationship

The one word that comes closest to embodying the personalist approach is "relationship." Solving difficult human problems often takes more than calculated advice—it often requires that we get involved in a personal way. To do this, we need a way of understanding the needs and values of those we're dealing with. But personal values are among the most private of human possessions. And, if those values are weak or immature, they can be even more hidden and fragile. How do we get the knowledge we need? We get it through our direct personal relationships.

Are human relationships some kind of mystical event, a topic reserved for sentimental poetry? Not at all. The capacity for developing personal relationships is a basic, universal human characteristic. It's the imaginative ability to see other people as more than just things.

When we observe a thing, we're mentally standing back, viewing from a distance. The experience of a personal relationship is different—it's a motion into another's deep privacy. This motion is active, and it's chosen. It occurs because it's accepted and encouraged on both sides.

Yet this motion isn't always easy or automatic. As we work to know another person as a unique individual, we always experience a resistance to our efforts. As Paul Weiss of the Catholic University points out in his brilliant work *Privacy*, the inner private self of each person is always active, it "pushes back." The essence of relationship, then, is motion and resistance. Still, if we're going to use this capacity in a practical way, we'll need to know more about it than that. If we're going to become experts at achieving meaningful relationships, we'll need to reflect deeply about what really happens when someone "lets us in."

Putting this kind of knowledge into words isn't easy, but it's worth the effort. Knowing more about what goes into a solid human relationship, we'll have a better chance of getting through when time is short or the obstacles are great. Also, if we understand how relationships should work, we'll have a better chance of fixing them when they don't.

One way to organize this knowledge is to describe what necessarily happens in a positive relationship. Following the lead of abnormal psychology, which analyzes disturbed relationships, we'll want to clearly understand strong, mature relationships. In the next few paragraphs we'll briefly describe four elements of a healthy personal relationship.

Openness. Entering into a positive relationship, our mental predisposition is openness, or receptivity. This is a desire and willingness to close the distance between ourselves and another person. At the heart of this attitude is an interest in knowing the other person, not changing him or her. This mind-set doesn't come easily to most of us, but it can be practiced and developed by conscious effort.

The opposite of openness is judgmentalism. The judgmental mind is interested more in labeling than knowing. It backs away from others into the security of abstractions. Remaining open, though, we offer to engage others' problems with them, willing to learn in the process.

Trust. The basic tone or atmosphere of a personal relationship is trust, a confidence that we won't be used impersonally. When people enter into a relationship of trust, they mutually imply that they won't use their knowledge for purely selfish reasons.

Trust is more than a passive willingness to go along, it actually encourages us to be independent, so we can accept the company of others without *needing* them impersonally, the way we need or use things. This isn't the kind of independence that says "I don't need anyone or anything." It says "I'm strong enough to get to know you without trying to get something out of you."

Vulnerability. An unavoidable condition that is accepted in our pursuit of a personal relationship is vulnerability. This is an acceptance of our own inner resistance to opening up, and a willingness to accept the risks of letting another in. Will the other person come to find that I'm not as valuable as they first thought me to be? Will that person find weakness in me that even I didn't realize was there? Will he or she make demands on me that I'd rather not take on?

Even vulnerability has its positive side. In our relationships with others we sometimes find strength in our mutual vulnerability. The example of another, overcoming his or her natural reluctance, can lead us to take greater risks than we otherwise might. The sense of vulnerability, originally a barrier, can become a bond.

Responsibility. The unavoidable result of a personal relationship is responsibility. This is a personally accepted obligation to stand with the other person in spite of the difficulties that doing so might cause for us.

Unlike social obligations, which arise from a social role, personal responsibility must be deeply and continuously chosen. Finding and accepting responsibility is something we do because we're free to do so, not because someone else says we have to. In a way, our responsibilities to others actually expand our personal freedom, even when they limit our external choices.

"Responding to" another, though, doesn't mean passively accepting his or her felt needs as valid or final. It does mean accepting those needs as *real* and being willing to engage them in a positive way. It also means continuing to be committed to that relationship even when it becomes difficult or awkward.

OUR PRACTICAL RESOURCES

Unfortunately, talking about personal relationships doesn't necessarily mean that we're capable of responding to real, live people. Ethics is finally a practical activity, one that is more interested in excellent, meaningful choices than in idealistic descriptions. In fact, in a personalist ethics, abstract theory should occupy only a small part of our attention. Even more important are our own practical resources, such as our abilities to listen, communicate, and understand. Studying these skills, and working to improve ourselves, is central to the personalist approach.

For example, listening is especially important if we're serious about getting to know people. Quality listening involves attending to what others are really trying to say, not just to their words. It's imaginative and creative. It tries to make the other person's thoughts, feelings, and experiences our own. Like reflection, it isn't judgmental—it's intrigued by what's new, not threatened by it.

Active listening can be a more powerful tool than anything technology can offer. Listening carefully, we sometimes appreciate what others are trying to say even before they do. Learning more about others' most positive values, we can help them find ways of expressing those values better than they could on their own.

Similarly, skilled communication can contribute as much to our healing efforts as any technical procedure we could master. Learning to express our perceptions clearly, we can often cut to the heart of the matter. We can keep others' attentions focused, helping them work more surely toward a successful answer.

Communicating can be done poorly or excellently. Arguing or giving advice is usually low quality communication, especially if we don't have the benefit of knowing the other person in a deeply personal way. More useful than advice can be the effort simply to describe a difficult situation, bringing it more clearly into full view. Where advice often signals an end to discussion, a summary indicates that we are looking for ways of getting more deeply involved.

Even our choice of vocabulary can affect our results. Technical words, so useful on the wards, can cut us off from those who have no reason to be fluent in this foreign language. Translating to our native tongue may take effort, but it can demonstrate that we're really interested in getting our message across.

Another personal skill that is invaluable in dealing with people is a sense of humor. More than just a gift for telling jokes, a real sense of humor helps us keep perspective in our lives. It doesn't belittle the serious feelings we have, but brings them out into the open and says that they're alright. When we're exhausted and ready to give up, a sense of humor renews our interest in working through to a positive solution.

Of course, these personal skills are complex; perfecting them isn't done overnight. But, without conscious effort, our abilities can easily go undeveloped. Even our simplest dealings with others can provide opportunities to expand and deepen our talents. Our personal strengths are really our ethical stock in trade. No matter how adept we are at analyzing human problems, we can't succeed unless we're able to work well with others as individuals. Learning to get through quickly and surely, we can be more confident from the start.

PERSONALISM AND THE ISSUES

Whenever an ethical theory is being discussed, inevitably the question comes up, "How does this system deal with abortion (or euthanasia, or any other general issue)?" Most theories retreat from these questions. Personalism doesn't. That's because the answers aren't really as difficult as people make them. Elective abortion *is* bad, it's wrong. So is active euthanasia. So is purposeful deception. These human choices are limiting—they don't, in and of themselves, express our deepest respect for human life.

But there's more. *Therapeutic* abortion is also wrong, as is *passive* euthanasia. And so is paternalism, human experimentation, and unequal care for different individuals. In fact, any choice that shows less than our full capacity for valuing people as unique and important is bad or evil.

However, that's still only part of the story—the rest is even more important. Being unable to even *consider* doing any of these things is also wrong, bad, or evil. If we've made up our minds, with no further room for thought, we've stopped listening to those who come to us for help and we've lost our fullest respect for human life.

We have to be able to deal with these problems without judgmentalism. We have to be able to get involved in the fullest way possible—and that means being open to the possibility that we could participate in any of these choices, and that such participation could even be a moral imperative, the only really right thing to do.

This idea is worth repeating. We should be willing to accept the idea that *some* occasion could arise when we would do any of these "evil" things and that such a choice could be truly moral and excellent. We should always be looking for that occasion and we should be terrified of ever coming across it.

Case 13

You live in Elephant Butte, Minnesota. You are the only physician within 150 miles. Mrs. N comes to you for a pregnancy test, then breaks into tears when you tell her that the test is positive. You know her, and you know that she is losing the battle of raising seven children with an alcoholic husband in the house. Indeed, it's Mr. N who staunchly forbids the use of birth control.

Mrs. N says that another child will simply be impossible for her. But she can't afford the trip to the city for an abortion, much less the procedure itself. Although you're technically able to perform abortions, you're morally opposed to them. Should you put your principles aside, or stand by them?

Perhaps Mrs. N's situation isn't the one that would lead us to sacrifice a human life—but, then again, maybe it is. If we don't look further into the human context here, we'll never know. We aren't saying to ourselves that abortion is okay, because it really isn't okay—we're saying that participating in an abortion *could* be our only meaningful response to a sad human condition.

But we can't change the fact that abortion, *any* kind of abortion, is wrong. Labeling it "therapeutic" doesn't make it somehow "good," and it doesn't take away our responsibility. The same is true of euthanasia. Calling it "passive" doesn't change the fact that we've chosen to hasten a human death.

If we're using soft-sounding words as insulation against what we're really doing, we're only fooling ourselves. Facing these issues *should* be difficult, each and every time we come across them. When we stop feeling the seriousness of what we're doing, we've lost something—we've lost our sensitivity to the importance of human life.

Doing an abortion should never be easy. Turning off life support should never be easy, either. We're all human, and we all make mistakes; we can't escape the chance that we're doing the wrong thing. But refusing to get involved with people's problems because we've made up our minds ahead of time is wrong, too. So we look at *all* the possibilities open to us, we make choices, and we accept responsibility for them.

Actually, for the personalist, nothing is really off limits. But this is hardly the same as saying that "anything goes." Our choices do matter. There's always a question of right and wrong, but the question isn't settled ahead of time. It's settled in the context of our own best and most mature values, and those of the people we're dealing with.

Of course, this doesn't mean that we shouldn't have personal beliefs or principles. Our personal ideals provide structure, they're the framework for our own search for meaning in life. But forcing these beliefs on others doesn't reinforce them, it weakens them. All of our other personal principles still need to be measured against a higher one—namely, our respect for the importance and dignity of the human person.

There may be times when we'll do things that go against our personal beliefs, because there's no other way to truly demonstrate our respect for people and their needs. But the opposite is also true: there will be times when we'll dig in our heels and take a stand—times when we won't go along with what others want us to do, no matter what anyone says.

Those are the times when weak or immature decisions are being made, and we know that better ones are possible. As personalists, we don't necessarily agree with the values of others, but we do accept those values as real and try to work with them. Our aim isn't to change others' values to match our own, but to participate in human decisions that are as meaningful as they can be.

In order to make this approach work, we've got to have a firm hold on our own personal values. Our values must be as mature and solid as we can make them. But we also have to be flexible enough to realize that our reflective work is never really finished. As we work with others, as we encounter new problems, we have to be ready to learn and grow.

HOW PERSONALISM WORKS: A SUMMARY

Preparation

1. Self-reflection: identifying our own values.

Getting the Observational Knowledge We Need

2. Identify the ethical or personal problem, as early as possible. Focus on the most pressing problems first.

3. Get the medical facts straight. Know the prognosis with and without treatment.

4. Identify the critical people. A single illness almost always affects several individuals.

Getting the Relational Knowledge

5. Listen. Get an understanding of the other's needs and values. Learn and profit from their experiences and insights. Communicate our own thoughts and concerns clearly.

6. Get an idea of the other person's potential for dealing with the problem. Try to locate unrecognized inner resources.

Doing the Ethical Work

7. Reflect again. Look for unique answers to difficult problems.

8. The easiest step: making a decision about what's best to do in this instance. These decisions are rarely, if ever, made alone or in advance.

9. Stay involved: look for opportunities to continue the work of healing.

Now let's try a more difficult case to test out this approach:

Case 14

Tom G. is sixteen years old. He has cystic fibrosis, and he's been hospitalized for what will probably be his last pneumonia. Even with adequate treatment, his respiratory status is steadily deteriorating. Tom is very bright and mature, and he knows that the end is near. He has asked that he not be subjected to CPR or mechanical ventilation, since he knows that they will only forestall the inevitable. He frequently brings up the issue of "death with dignity."

His mother, though, has made it clear that she wishes Tom to be "full code." She believes that there are still many good months in store for him, and she's afraid of wasting them. She also points out that Tom is a minor, and so her wishes are controlling. Tom's father remains silent on the subject.

If the answer to this dilemma seems easy or obvious, then we're missing something. Whatever we decide to do, it isn't likely to be easy. But, difficult or not, decisions must be made. So what will we do?

Even though this is a difficult case, it's an everyday one; a personalist ethics takes it in stride. Our goal isn't to decide what to do *to* Tom, but to decide how best to work *with* the various people involved, without compromising our own deepest values. To accomplish this we have to learn more about their perceptions, needs, values, and potential for growth.

Tom's mother has clearly established herself as a patient, even though she may not know it. She may be even more deeply injured by Tom's disease than he is. She's an obvious target for our efforts to listen and understand. In fact, she may be more in need of our attention than Tom himself.

As healers, people like Tom's mother aren't the enemy, even when they don't agree with us. It's crucial that we prevent the situation from becoming one of choosing up sides. Our *only* real adversary in this case is Tom's cystic fibrosis—the people involved, all of them, are victims.

After we've inventoried the patients (probably including ourselves and the other staff members on the list), we'll want to inventory the resources. Usually our best resources are our own personal skills and those of the others involved.

Tom, being mature beyond his years, and apparently blessed with an uncommon degree of common sense, may be a great ally to us in finding a successful solution. He may be a very healing person himself, and he may be able to help us in the initial task of reaching the other family members. In becoming involved in a positive way, he may also find his last days to be much more meaningful than they would otherwise be.

If we're attentive, if we work hard, and if we have a little luck, we may discover the reason why Tom's mother is so irrationally determined that he must live. But figuring her out isn't the same as understanding her. Our final goal isn't to change her, but to help her deal with the realities of this situation in the best way she can. At the same time we need to help Tom deal with the realities of the situation (including his mother) in the best way he's able.

It should be apparent by now that the personalist approach is less interested in making the situation fit our preconceived notion of what's right, than in helping those who are ill to make the most positive choices they can. Even though we may have clear and strict moral standards by which we live, forcing these standards on other people isn't part of living a moral life.

What would be most wrong in this case would be to polarize the case further, creating more conflict than existed originally. What would be most right would be to understand the individuals involved, and use their personal strengths to counter the human damage being done by the cystic fibrosis. Also "right" is a personal commitment to stay involved even after Tom's death, continuing the work of healing wherever we can.

Using a personalist approach, we don't have to have all the answers before we start playing the game. There's a reliable way for us to get the answers we need as we go. That way is personal relationship. Still, the real test of a theory isn't how nice it sounds over coffee, but what it can do for us when we need help. In the next chapter we're going to translate some of these theoretical ideas into more practical tools for problem solving.

8 Putting Theory into Practice

In this book we've often referred to the needs and values of others. But most of us come to ethics with a personal need of our own: a need to have greater confidence in the quality of our choices. We want to feel good about our involvement with others. We want to feel that what we do really counts. This is a natural human need, and a very meaningful one. So in this chapter we're going to be more concrete and pragmatic. We're going to show how ethical reasoning can help solve problems.

Even though the model used here is personalist philosophy, it isn't necessary to choose personalism, or any other theory, in order to act ethically. In fact, in order to begin, all we need are the following:

·a firm conviction that quality really matters,
·an unshakable sense of respect for people,
·an interest in reflecting honestly about the meaning of life,
·an openness to new ideas, and
·a determination to stay involved even when the going is tough.

If we have these qualities, we're ready to start, if we don't, all the theories in the world won't help us.

A WORD OF CAUTION

When we're looking at ethical choices, it's assumed that we already have the technical information straight. This means that we're reasonably sure of the diagnosis, that we have a clear idea of the prognosis, both with and without treatment, and that we're aware of appropriate treatments. If we haven't answered the medical questions, it's a little early to tackle the ethical ones.

Case 15

Mr. P was a hugely obese diabetic. One night he came to the emergency room looking quite ill, and promptly stopped breathing. A full arrest situation ensued, and his heart was resuscitated. Since he had no regular doctor, a young physician from the Emergency Room's on-call list was assigned.

This is Mr. P's third hospital day. He's on a ventilator, his pneumonia is being treated with the finest of antibiotics, his vital signs are stable—but he's not waking up. His EEG shows no ordered activity, and he's having constant fine seizures in spite of medication. The question now is whether mechanical ventilation ought to be continued. No family members or close friends are available to help with the decision.

The working diagnosis here is anoxic encephalopathy. If that's correct, the prognosis after three days is dismal. But are there other possibilities? Could he have taken an overdose? Could he have meningitis? The reversible causes of coma need to be excluded before we presume that the situation is hopeless. Even though the likelihood is low, the stakes are high.

It's not alright to withdraw support from Mr. P simply because we haven't been thorough in pursuing a diagnosis, or because we're unaware of effective treatments for his disease. This doesn't mean that we should go to ridiculous lengths to rule out obscure problems, and it doesn't mean that we should try every remote possibility for a cure. It does mean that we should perform our technical job in a reasonable fashion.

THE PRACTICAL APPROACH: ASKING THE RIGHT QUESTIONS

When we're finally down to grappling with the ethical problems in a real case, what we *don't* need is a huge heap of theoretical questions. In fact, if a co-worker comes to us for help with a difficult case, and we simply pour forth a litany of conflicting questions, we'll certainly deserve the disgusted sigh we receive.

Still, asking the right questions at the right time can be extremely useful. The key is to keep our questions simple and direct. In this section, we'll outline some questions that can put us back on track when we're not sure what's right to do. In fact, the majority of ethical dilemmas can be solved by answering just one or two of them:

·Who are the patients here?

·How well do I know them?

·What do I have to offer?

·Is there more healing to be done?

WHO ARE THE PATIENTS HERE?

This is an exceptionally useful question, one that is worth returning to again and again. It can reveal the source of our problem when things aren't working out, but we're not sure why. It can also help us recognize more opportunities for healing than appear on the surface.

Case 16

An elderly patient, Mr. H, is admitted with weight loss. His barium enema shows a large cecal carcinoma. As the third-year medical student on the surgery service, your job is to present the idea of surgery to him. You're a little lukewarm about it, though, since his severe chronic lung disease makes postoperative complications almost a certainty.

Mr. H, unsurprisingly, says that he wants nothing further done, that he's "lived a full life." His daughter, however, is adamant that surgery be done. She says that her father is "obviously depressed," and that if you don't take him to the operating room, she'll have her lawyers deal with you.

To make matters worse, the attending, an internist, is convinced that experimental chemotherapy ought to be tried. Your argument with him over the matter doesn't seem to have improved anything. The nursing staff is growing more and more uncomfortable with what's going on. They think that Mr. H's wishes should be respected above all.

Who's affected by Mr. H's illness? He is, of course. But clearly his daughter is, too, and she seems to be having even more trouble with the situation than he is. The medical team is at odds, and the nursing staff is being dragged down as well. One cancer, lots of patients.

Are all of these people really ill? Yes they are. If something isn't done, they're all headed for more symptoms in the future. They'll have trouble with their health, difficulties at home, and their work will suffer. They'll lose a bit of their self-confidence and they'll enjoy life less. Pretending that there's no problem won't solve a thing.

The daughter and the attending physician want to do things to Mr. H that he doesn't want. Are they the enemy? Are they our problem? Not at all. People aren't diseases. In fact, in the case of Mr. H, everyone's trying to help, but some of them aren't able to, because of their own problems with the case.

The person with a terminal illness isn't always the one who's most devastated by its effects. Sometimes it's a relative, a friend, or a family member. It may even be a staff member whose personal resources are being pushed to their limit. Identifying these people, and their needs, can be crucial if we're to accomplish something positive.

When we're making out our tentative list of patients, it's usually wise to put ourselves on the list automatically. If we're surrounded by well-meaning people who are struggling with an ethical problem, it should mean that we're having trouble, too.

HOW WELL DO I KNOW THEM?

Once we've identified the people affected by an illness, our job has just begun. The really critical work involves coming to know them in a personal way.

There will be times when we've known the important people for years, and we understand their values very clearly. Supporting them and their decisions comes easily. In effect, we've done our homework before the last minute. Other times, such as in the Emergency Room, we're dealing with strangers, and there's no time for long conferences. These situations are also fairly straightforward, since our only real choice is to support the value of human life.

The really difficult cases, though, are the ones in which all the pieces don't seem to fit. This happens when we expect someone to make a certain choice, and they surprise us by choosing something else.

Case 17

Mrs. V, seventy-four years old, is an ex-alcoholic who's always been a difficult patient. She's been demanding and attention seeking in the past, and has always needed pills for everything. Fortunately, she's never been very sick. Now things are different. She was recently diagnosed as having a fairly aggressive lymphoma—the primary tumor arising from the cervical lymph nodes.

The tumor has continued to grow in spite of chemotherapy. Now it's beginning to cause some airway problems. There's a living will in her chart, and earlier she said that she didn't want to undergo CPR if there wasn't much to gain. Now, though, she's not so sure. She thinks that she wants everything done, so that "the chemotherapy can have a chance to work." Her husband has been in favor of aggressive treatment all along. You wish they'd make up their minds.

People aren't always consistent. Sometimes they say one thing, but later say something completely different. Sometimes their choices are contradictory or confusing. This doesn't mean that they are thoughtless, but only that they are human. Our knowledge of others, like their own knowledge of themselves, is always a process, never a completed fact.

We need to be flexible in our approach. As Paul Weiss points out, there is "considerable slippage" between what people appear to be on the surface, and what they are inwardly. Our goal in knowing others is to reach the inner person, not to force them to follow our expectations.

In the case of Mrs. V, her indecisiveness isn't necessarily a sign of inadequacy, but it is a clue to the fact that we don't know her as well as we thought. Is that her fault or ours? Actually it's neither, it's merely a signal that more work needs to be done.

What are Mrs. V's deepest values? Apparently, we made some assumptions about her values based on her signing a living will. But why did she really sign it? Because her husband signed one? Because it seemed like the fashionable thing to do? Or because she wished to express some deep personal values, reflectively and thoughtfully held? If her reasons for signing the living will were strong and mature, perhaps all she needs now is a little support to carry it through. If her reasons for signing it were superficial or weak, it may be too late for her to do better. If that's so, then we may find ourselves supporting choices that we ourselves might not make.

As we get to know others, then, we're not just trying to "figure them out." Instead, we're trying to help them find inner resources that can help them at a critical time in their lives. This requires an openness to their actual values, whatever they may be. It also requires an interest in appreciating what they're realistically capable of, their unique personal promise.

Maybe Mrs. V won't be able to do what she imagined herself doing, now that the problem is real. Even so, maybe she'll still be able to make some real progress in exploring the meaning in her life. Regardless of what she finally chooses, we can hope that her last days are meaningful and worth living. If they are, then she's living ethically.

Case 18

You're a technician in a busy dialysis unit. One day, Mrs. M (who's one of your favorite patients), fails to keep her appointment for routine dialysis. Fearing that she may be too ill to come in for treatment, you call her at home. She answers the phone, and explains to you that she's simply "tired of it all," and that she's decided to go off dialysis. You point out to her the seriousness of the decision she's making, and she agrees. She thanks you for your concern and hangs up.

Although this lady's decision *might* be reasonable, we can't tell much about the quality of her decision unless we have more information. Spending a little time getting that information can be the key to finding a meaningful answer. Perhaps Mrs. M is depressed because of something unrelated to her illness. Perhaps she's angry about something said to her by a staff member, but is misinterpreting her feelings. Perhaps she's tired of being a financial drain on her family, even though they don't feel the same. Then again, this may be a perfectly valid decision that she's arrived at after deep reflection. Perhaps this choice fits the pattern of the other life choices which she's made in the past. The only way to get the information we need is to talk to Mrs. M.

Gut level instincts about the quality of these types of important decisions aren't good enough. Standing back to analyze the "logic" of these choices can mislead us, too. Abstract reasoning often falls short in solving human problems—the answers that work for one person may not fit another at all.

Is it always wrong to pass up life-sustaining treatment? Of course not. Can there be wrong or limited reasons for making the decision to embrace death? Certainly. Until we know more about the reasons behind Mrs. M's decision, we don't have enough to to go by.

WHAT DO I HAVE TO OFFER?

Once we've identified the players, and we know their strengths and weaknesses, we're ready to start working with the ethical choices. Again, the measure of our actions and choices is how well they demonstrate our respect for people, their personal needs, and their personal values.

Chiefly, what we have to offer others is the fruit of our own best reflective efforts, our most solid and mature values. When we believe that others are making strong, meaningful decisions, we can give them our encouragement and support. We can be there. These occasions are a privilege—our greatest reward for personal involvement.

When we believe that weak or immature decisions are being made, though, it's not quite so easy. However, if all we have to offer is a lecture on right and wrong, we might as well go for a walk. When people are in trouble, they need to find ways to access their deepest personal strengths—they rarely need the benefit of our abstract opinions.

Case 19

Gary is eleven years old. He was found to have leukemia three months ago—bone marrow biopsy showed it to be a fairly poorly differentiated tumor, most likely myelocytic. Because the prognosis wasn't good, the attending oncologist decided that strenuous chemotherapy wouldn't be appropriate unless there was at least a fair response to more moderate treatment.

Unfortunately, Gary's initial response to treatment was poor. The staff has grown very fond of Gary, but now he is clearly dying; probably only a few days are left. All of a sudden, the oncologist reverses himself, saying that he wants to try an experimental regimen. The staff is shocked. They hate the thought of making Gary's last days miserable, with nausea, painful IV medications, and frequent needle sticks. Gary is beginning to look like a sad, emaciated, trapped animal.

It appears that Gary's oncologist is a patient along with him, and so is the nursing staff. As one of the staff members, you feel like choosing up sides: suddenly, the oncologist is more the enemy than the leukemia. Pretty soon, Gary is caught in the middle, and no one has enough energy left to really be there for him. At this point, we've at least identified the patients.

Why this sudden change on the part of the oncologist? Is he using the order sheet to keep a safe distance from Gary's death? Is he "doing something" so that he won't feel quite so inadequate, in spite of the fact that it's Gary who will suffer? Or has he come across some promising new studies, and now thinks that there really is a good chance for Gary to live?

Before we can do much to help, we'll have to know more about this doctor's reasons for moving ahead with chemotherapy. Approaching him may be difficult, especially if we suspect that he's acting out of personal weakness. But, like it or not, it's got to be done.

In this case, it turns out that he has burned the midnight oil a bit, and has turned up some solid evidence to support a new protocol. Unfortunately, he's not a very good communicator, and he has neglected to share the new information with the staff. His motives are correct, but his "people" skills are a little weak. If that's so, perhaps all that's necessary to restore the health of the team is a staff conference. If the nurses know that they are fighting a battle with at least a small chance of success, they may be able to renew their determination to fight the leukemia.

Now let's change the story a bit. Let's say that our first suspicions about the oncologist are correct, that he's hiding behind the order sheet so that he won't have to feel Gary's death and his own frustration so intensely. Is there something we can do in that case?

If he's a well-meaning fellow, he'll want to know more about the problems of the nursing staff. Simply opening the door and pointing him in the right direction is all we need to do. He'll learn that, even though it's fairly easy to write orders, it isn't always so easy to carry them through. He'll see that writing those orders also makes him responsible to those who must put them into action.

If he's not a well-meaning fellow, and he says that he can't be bothered by any of this "psycho-social stuff," we'll have to deal with him and move on. A meeting with the hospital's medical director might be a good idea. But refocusing the staff's attention on Gary's needs is still the most valuable, meaningful thing we can do.

When we're trying to decide what we have to offer, we're taking an inventory of what we perceive as the human assets or strengths of the situation. Taking stock of the personal resources available usually can give us some good ideas about what's best to do. Remember, though, that we can't tally our assets and liabilities until we have accurate knowledge about the people involved—assumptions won't do.

Again, the patient is often one of our best resources. When a patient is in a terminal condition, he or she is often "declared dead" ahead of time. In fact, the dying often have a great deal to share, if we're willing to use them as a resource. Making the effort to involve them in what's going on can also make their last important days more worth living.

IS THERE MORE HEALING TO BE DONE?

Before we put a difficult case aside and move on, it's a good idea to ask this question. In effect, it returns us to the first question we asked above: Are there still important human needs that haven't been met? Are there people we've overlooked, because their needs didn't seem as pressing as others'? Are there people who will be ill in the future because of what's gone on—and is there something we can do now to avoid that? This is preventative care, ethical style.

In some situations, asking this question is really just icing on the cake. By participating in really excellent decision making, we've averted the worst problems that could come up. In other cases, though, studying this question is all we have to offer, since circumstances haven't allowed us to achieve as much as we might have hoped. For example, in the case of Tom in the previous chapter, what finally happened was considerably short of ideal, even though the team did everything it could. After Tom's death, though, the case wasn't really closed.

There was still the problem of Tom's mother. Would she later realize what she put Tom through and feel guilty? Would Tom's father later blame himself for not being more actively involved? Would the nursing staff be less functional because of what went on? Being aware of these potential problems could give us a head start on healing those who were injured by Tom's sad end.

In fact, in almost every case example in this book, there are hidden opportunities for healing that we would probably miss unless we were looking. Training ourselves to watch for these possibilities for involvement can make our own efforts more effective and more meaningful.

Asking this question basically returns us to the idea of quality. It reminds us that being available even after the "big" choices have been made is part of ethics. Accepting full responsibility for our involvement with others doesn't really limit us—it opens doors that would otherwise remain tightly locked.

9   Social Ethics (Politics)

Early in the book we introduced a variety of controversial issues like euthanasia, truth-telling, and genetic engineering. Now we're going to look at these kinds of problems a little more closely. Some readers may be thinking that we've saved the best for last. Actually, we've put this chapter at the end because social ethics, for healers, is far less important than personal ethics.

Personal ethics involves reflectively building a strong set of internalized values, and applying those values to the choices we make in our dealings with others. Its goal is really to make our lives as meaningful as possible.

Social ethics looks at human problems in a much more abstract and distant way. It tries to develop general answers to common ethical problems, so that society's laws can also reflect strong and mature values.

Is social policy part of the job of ethics? Actually it is, and it's even thought by some to be the most important work of ethics. In this chapter, we'll put social ethics into perspective, then we'll look at how a personalist might analyze some of the common ethical issues of health care.

THE DIFFERENCE BETWEEN PERSONAL AND SOCIAL ETHICS

For individuals, ethics is a personal search for values that work, ones that have lasting meaning. Ethicists are people who help us recognize and develop this inner side of ourselves.

There's an offshoot of ethics, though, that focuses on ethical issues taken abstractly. This is politics (going back to the original Greek meaning of the word). Politicians are people whom we've elected to help us deal with ethical issues on a larger, social level. They devise morally "good" ways of solving social problems.

The following diagram lists the kinds of activities which occur under the broad definition of ethics:

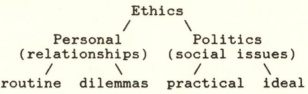

Personal ethics looks at how we deal with others, both in ordinary situations, and in unusual ones (dilemmas). Politics tries to develop answers to general questions. It suggests how things might be in a perfect world, as well as the solutions that are most likely to work in the real world.

Which activity is more important? Both certainly have their place. But politics relies heavily on personal ethics to help it move in a morally good direction. The quality of our society's laws depends on the reflective insight and strong moral values of those who devise them. Personal ethics, on the other hand, doesn't rely on politics for anything.

Moreover, for those who work professionally with others, simply following the law may not be enough. There may be occasions where the law doesn't anticipate an important and valid human need—and we may have to go beyond its minimum requirements. Or there may be occasions where, after reflecting deeply on the dictates of the law, we find it morally lacking. In those cases, the law may need to be challenged in order to grow.

For the purposes of this book, then, the more important activities appear on the left-hand side of the above diagram. But as citizens in this society, in which each individual is expected to offer an informed opinion by means of a vote, politics is important too.

Actually, carrying this idea a little further, each of us is a politician. Each of us has a real stake in the future of our society and the expression of its most deeply held values. When we work to develop general opinions about abstract social issues we are mentally "doing" politics.

Trying to find answers that work well for everyone is more than challenging—it's next to impossible. Recognizing this, our governmental system relies on the individual application of laws through the judiciary. This one-to-one work is so important that the judicial system has the final say in whether a law is socially (and ethically) acceptable.

Even though it's very difficult to devise ideal laws, it's work that can't be ignored. Our society still needs policies and guidelines in order to function smoothly. Social regulations provide structure and education. They help us avoid the trap of having to re-invent the wheel every day. Laws also keep the small percentage of the population that is unscrupulous from victimizing the rest of us.

Is it useless, then, to discuss moral issues abstractly? Not at all. Tackling these issues can help us test our ideas and values. If our opinions are solicited by those whom we've elected (and if our ideas are sound), we may be able to make a contribution. But having strong opinions doesn't mean that our personal ethical work is done. In fact, it doesn't necessarily mean that it's even begun.

THE APPROACH TO SOCIAL ISSUES: SOME GENERAL OBSERVATIONS

Our Ethical Priorities

Abstract issues can be quite a distraction if we haven't yet put our responsibilities to individuals in proper perspective. It makes little sense to spend our time on general questions if our personal values and choices are weak or immature.

Debate over the "rightness" of our opinions is, at best, a very dilute form of ethics. In fact, it's quite possible to have excellent opinions about a variety of issues, yet be surrounded by a personal life that is in a shambles. On the other hand, if our personal values are strong and our priorities are mature, our relationships *will* be solid and meaningful—our personal world *will* be successful.

In the long run, learning to argue our opinions effectively doesn't provide us with the skills we'll need to work closely with people. It's important to remember that ethical problems don't really exist as ideas: they come into being only when an actual person experiences a problem. In the world of ethics, involvement is more important than debate.

From the personalist point of view, this fact is central and bears repetition: human problems don't exist abstractly. Until a real person encounters a problem, it doesn't exist. Looked at in this way, there really are no social issues, only personal issues that come up repeatedly. Further, whenever an individual faces a difficult personal choice, there's always a very real and specific context, namely that person's past experience, present needs, and continuing values. If ethical excellence is our goal, we can't avoid the difficult task of trying to understand problems as they exist in their human context.

An Historical Perspective

As we pointed out in Chapter 1, technology is at the root of many of our ethical problems, especially the general social ones. But technology isn't going to go away—we have to learn to live with it in a productive and sensible way.

A few historical observations are in order. First, what we *can* do, we probably *will* do. Over and over again our society has shown a tendency to move forward with technological "progress," regardless of the inherent dangers. Our rapid movement into the nuclear age is an excellent example. The point here is that it's unrealistic simply to say that we shouldn't proceed with a new technology. Whether we should or not, we probably will. More reasonable is an effort to develop ways in which we can handle new technology in a life-enhancing and beneficial way. In other words, helping us chart a positive and meaningful course is what ethics is about, rather than just standing back and saying "I told you so."

Another general observation that is clear to the student of history is that nearly every new technological advance in our society has been quickly commercialized. This can be dangerous in that the only controls at work are economic ones: "If it will sell, let's be the first to sell it."

Ethics certainly encourages us to be a bit more thoughtful in our approach, and health care ethics is especially conservative in this regard. Although health care is a biologically oriented job, it's different from breeding domestic animals or farming. Commodity-ism must be watched for and checked—by legal means if all others fail. Protecting ourselves from ourselves is one of the ways that the legal system can further our best ethical intentions.

Finally, we should try to avoid what the Existentialists call the "frightened flight from death." Health care ethics commonly deals with issues of life and death. Our focus should be steadfastly on the quality and meaning of life, not just its duration. Admittedly, none of us is completely comfortable with the prospect of death and its manifest unknowns. But we shouldn't allow this insecurity to guide our decisions in an unbalanced way.

PERSONALISM AND THE APPROACH TO SOCIAL ISSUES

When we confront social ethical issues, it's important that we have a theoretical guide to direct us. "Gut-level" instincts about what's right have only a minor role in ethics. The authors have chosen the personalist approach, which has limitations like any other, but we've seen it work for us. The reader may choose an entirely different approach.

Regardless of our theoretical leanings, the real key to success in dealing with social issues is honesty in evaluating our results, and a willingness to admit the limitations of our thinking. This rarely means giving up and standing quietly at the sidelines, but it usually does involve careful and open listening to the thoughts and insights of others.

Within the framework of personalism, one question is central: How can we structure our society so that we demonstrate our respect for individuals as fully as possible? Or, restated in a retrospective way: Do the laws of our society demonstrate respect for people as fully as they possibly can?

In order to answer these questions, we need insight into the values of the people who live in society with us. We need to be able to recognize weak or immature values for what they are, and to have some skill at helping others find and use more meaningful values. As we suggested earlier, we don't try to learn about the values of others in order to do what they want. Pleasing others in a superficial way isn't our goal. We work to know people and their values so that we can be sure that the best possible choices are made, considering the human and external circumstances.

There may be times when people want us to support them in weak, immature choices—and we may have to ask more of them. Then again, people may surprise us by doing better than we ourselves could in a similar situation, and we find ourselves learning from them and thanking them for letting us participate in their choice.

When we learn about people and their values, our attention should remain fixed on excellence, which we've defined for ourselves by deep and thoughtful reflection. We don't always demonstrate respect for people by respecting their individuality. We show our respect by helping them achieve the best they can given the circumstances and their own personal resources.

THE ISSUES THEMSELVES

In Chapter 5 we looked at a variety of complex ethical issues, and it seemed as if the more we looked at them, the more complicated they became. How does personalism see specific issues? Does it just give us more impossible questions, or does it put us closer to meaningful answers? In this section we'll demonstrate how a personalist might approach some of these common problems. The same principles can be used to deal with most other general ethical problems as well.

Abortion

The debate surrounding this question is largely artificial; the facts are reasonably straightforward. The embryo or fetus, *left alone*, holds the promise of personhood. This is particularly true after twelve weeks' gestation, but it's still true from the moment of conception on. If we don't interfere, the majority of fetuses will go on to become people, as capable of finding meaning and value in life as any of us.

Viewed in this way, abortion is simply wrong. But this is only part of the story. As we discussed in the previous chapter, it's also wrong to have our minds made up in advance, with no further room for considering the needs and values of real people. The conflict, then, is this: fetuses have the promise of becoming people, but the women who carry them are people too. To act in a mature ethical fashion, we can't ignore the needs of either group.

The personalist approach is this: the fetus is a person, or at least a being that holds the promise of personhood. Taking the life of this being is wrong, since it goes against our fundamental respect for the value of human life. But failing to listen to the needs of the mother who hasn't the personal resources to raise a child for eighteen or twenty years is also wrong.

The resolution is this. Abortion ought to be avoided as the serious evil it is. But we must remain open to the possibility that the needs of a real person could be so compelling that abortion would be the only positive answer to a difficult human situation. In other words, we should resist abortion internally, but continue to listen to the needs of those who see no other recourse.

"Resisting abortion," though, isn't something we can do mechanically, by making it especially difficult to obtain one. It means being thoughtful and reflective each and every time the problem comes up. It means making an effort to understand the whole human situation in every case, and to take it *very* seriously every time.

If we do this, we will encounter cases where abortion is the only thoughtful answer in an imperfect world. When those cases arise, they will be sad ones, but ones that can't be wished away. Those are the days when our ethical thinking is put to its sorest test.

As to society's role, there must be a clear effort to help those who are confronting this difficult choice. The mother needs to reflect on her values and the possibilities open to her, and the physician or technician needs to have a firm grasp on positive, life-enhancing values. If these needs are ignored, the inner damage to those individuals may not surface immediately, but it will almost always appear.

In such an important area, society's obligation goes far beyond permitting or prohibiting, especially since it's clear from history that abortions will be done. Society needs to work to provide a context in which matters of life or death are dealt with delicately and with the wisdom they deserve. This duty can only be discharged where there is ongoing and substantial education for those who touch this difficult problem.

Defectives

To some, the child whose IQ is severely limited is defective. Once we begin comparing people quantitatively, though, we enter some very dangerous ethical territory. In fact, all of us are, by various standards, "defective." So where's the cutoff, where does "normal" end and "defective" begin; and how do we make measurements so accurate that we can trust human life to them?

Actually, our humanity isn't something that can be expressed in numbers. What sets us apart as humans is our ability to find meaning in life, our ability to bring our own personal values to an otherwise quite mechanical world. People are creative centers of valuing. The numerical size of their IQs means very little.

For the personalist, a person is a being capable of finding meaning and value in life, regardless of his or her appearance, intellect, or ability to live independently. The person who finds meaning and value in life is *fully* a person and deserves respect.

On the other hand, the infant who is unlikely to ever be capable of valuing, of finding meaning in life and relationship, is truly defective. If we have the means to bring out these qualities through our technical intervention, then no effort should be spared. If it's unlikely that our intervention will make a difference, then we should use our resources elsewhere.

Unfortunately, once we begin our work to restore the damaged infant, it's difficult to stop. We become emotionally involved, we're driven by our hopes. So, it's important to reevaluate our progress in such cases periodically. The fact that we've undertaken a project certainly doesn't guarantee its success. (This is discussed further below.)

Euthanasia

As personalists, our highest regard isn't for the duration of life, but for its meaning and quality. In fact, people often find great opportunities for growth in their final days, and that growth can be every bit as significant as any that went before. Even the person who has lost many of his or her fundamental abilities can find new ways of touching and appreciating the meaning of life.

As healers, our efforts should be steadfastly aimed at enriching the content of the lives we touch. Helping others find the inner resources to deal creatively with their problems, new or old, is part of the job of healing. The number of obstacles in the path may indicate how hard our job will be, but it doesn't always dictate the outcome.

There's a sobering finality to the fact of death, and its presence should always cause us to look reflectively at the substance and potential of life. Even for those of us who are quite religious, death suggests a loss of potential for being more than we are; it's an irrevocable loss of our human promise.

This fact is so important that for the personalist, the traditional distinction between active and passive euthanasia has little substance. Withholding treatment that could extend life destroys human promise just as surely as does the lethal injection. The hastening of death, when it could be delayed, is always a very serious matter.

Unfortunately, traditional ethics has taught us to think of passive euthanasia, the withholding of treatment, as generally "okay." Telling ourselves that we're simply "letting nature take its course," we try to convince ourselves that we're no longer responsible for what's happening. This isn't so. We form relationships, we make choices, and the responsibility is ours. Nature doesn't make choices, it doesn't have responsibility. When we choose not to treat, we *choose*—the responsibility is ours.

What lulls us into this false sense of security is the fact that we sometimes mislabel cases as passive euthanasia when they really aren't. This occurs when the ability to find meaning in life has *already* been irrevocably lost due to disease or accident. When we withhold treatment in such cases, this isn't euthanasia at all. When only biological functions remain, and basic human functions are gone, then the person has already been lost.

We can't generalize from these cases, where we have nothing to offer, to cases in which setbacks have occurred, but the person is basically intact, with the ability to bring values to life and find meaning there. In these cases, the withdrawal of support isn't substantially different from the active welcoming of death.

The choice to allow death to come to a thinking, valuing person, then, isn't one that can be made easily, and it certainly can never be made unilaterally. The feeling that "I would never want to live like that" means nothing. It is only in the context of a personal relationship that a choice as serious as hastening death can be made.

Does all this mean that active euthanasia, the choice to intervene so that death can come more swiftly, is always wrong? Not at all. There are cases where such a choice might express the best that mankind can bring to life. The real point is that *all* cases where death is allowed are truly serious.

Euthanasia, when it represents taking "the easy way out" is simply a representation of human weakness. The call to participate in such an enterprise is less than an honor. Our goal is to help others find meaning in life. There may be times, though, when the choice to die is truly a representation of human strength—a conscious assent to human freedom and promise. This can only occur where there has been deep reflection on the meaning of life itself.

In the end, active euthanasia, to the personalist, carries the same serious impact as passive euthanasia, no more, no less. Can euthanasia (active or passive) ever be a meaningful ethical choice? Certainly. Could it ever be an ordinary event? Never.

Society's role in euthanasia, like that of abortion, goes far beyond simply allowing or disallowing. The responsibility to educate is critical. If euthanasia is to be practiced in our society, it should be done within the context of mature ethical reflection and meaningful choice. Providing the educational raw materials for good choices is something society can help with.

Ordinary versus Extraordinary Means

This is another distinction that can lead us toward some very fuzzy thinking and insubstantial choices. In practice, the boundary between ordinary and extraordinary is just too vague, too dependent on circumstance, to be of much real use.

When we're confronting illness, we choose the best tools to counter the damage we find. There are times when our resources are clearly up to the task of restoring an individual to a meaningful, or at least a potentially meaningful, life. In these cases, we simply use whatever is at our disposal.

There are other times where we have nothing to offer in a technical sense—the damage is simply too severe. Using our most expensive and dangerous tools is pointless when there's nothing to gain. Again, these choices are fairly clear-cut.

The really difficult problems arise for most of us when we begin trying to save or restore an individual, but find that we're not up to the task. We're doing our best, but we're losing out. In these cases, we might agonize about what's ordinary and what's extraordinary, but this kind of internal debate is usually more distressing than helpful.

It is more productive to realize that each choice we make is remade on an ongoing basis, usually daily. We choose to turn on the ventilator, and we choose to turn it on again every day. When the ventilator is no longer offering anything to our patient, we don't really choose to turn it off at all—we simply choose not to turn it on any more.

This is much more than another semantic distinction. It's an acceptance of the fact that each of our choices is a continuous expression of our ability to choose. Each day, actually each minute, is an opportunity for us to bring our most mature values to life. What we've chosen before is part of our history, but it doesn't control us.

Once we've chosen to use the ventilator, is it alright to turn it off again? When the ventilator no longer serves to sustain a meaningful life, it simply makes no sense to choose it. So we stop using it.

What about the powerful antibiotics? When they are holding the pneumonia in check, but the patient will never be able to live meaningfully again, do we need to continue treating the pneumonia? No, when the situation becomes clear to us, we stop choosing to use that ineffective treatment.

But what about the IV fluids—is it alright to turn them off? Actually, there's no difference between the fluids and the ventilator, if neither has the ability to do what we want—namely, to restore a person to a meaningful life. Are there other ways of making a person comfortable once the fluids have been stopped? Yes there are, and we can choose to use those methods instead.

Regardless of the situation, the key lies in reevaluating what we've done on a frequent basis. Each day that we allow an order to stand, we've rechosen it. If it's working then it's "ordinary"; if it's not, then it has become "extraordinary" and we stop it. If we're not sure, we choose to continue another day, until we're more sure of what results our choices are bringing about.

THE ISSUE NONE OF US REALLY WANTS TO FACE: OUR GLOBAL RESPONSIBILITIES

Our world has become so small that people at all levels of our society travel across the globe. Of course, we usually go to popular resorts and cities, not to Calcutta or Bangladesh. But we *could* go to those terrible places if we wanted to. Even if we never leave home, we can't avoid being bombarded with visions of worlds beyond our own. We see the ghetto and the hopelessness that sets the tempo there. We read about the plight of the poorer nations of the world, and about the children who starve there as we read.

We can't help but ask ourselves, are those people less important than the ones who live next door, simply because we don't know them by name? Does it really make sense to agonize for days or weeks over a person in an ICU bed whose EEG shows minimal activity, whose life has effectively ended, while thousands of people starve to death in the same period?

These are difficult questions. They raise the issue of our larger responsibilities. If it's important to develop ethical policies toward those in other parts of our nation, how about the people in nations across the world? Is *my* child so much more important than the other children of the world that it really makes no difference if they live or die?

"It's our government's responsibility to see that these people are helped. That's what we pay taxes for." But we can't escape two final facts: we *know* the job's not being done, and we know that it's "do-able." Are we finally responsible? If the institutions we empower to carry out these important tasks aren't up to the job, is it alright to give up?

The problem is even more complicated than that, though. Our goal in most of our social and global outreach hasn't been to understand others, but to change them. We've become societal bulldozers. Unfortunately, most people don't want to be bulldozed, even if it means that they will be fed. They want to be respected for what they are.

People in many countries have rejected our help because the price is too high. Even if they want help, they still want their traditions and beliefs respected and appreciated. They want to be valued for what they are, not indoctrinated and used for political purposes. Can we somehow learn to help out of respect, not out of utility?

Even if we pass that first hurdle, can we stick to the job as long as it takes to earn those peoples' trust? Can we build a school and staff it until suspicions fade? If our goals are too short-sighted and self-serving, what thanks do we really deserve?

Our system was founded with a heavy, almost unbalanced emphasis on individual freedom. In a global society that is shrinking, this doesn't work. "Doing our own thing" while others starve supports a value that is limited and basically immature. Expecting others to be like us in order to earn our support isn't what ethics is about, either.

The personalist, thinking globally, looks for opportunities to learn and grow, not just opportunities to get ahead. The fundamental guide is respect for the concrete value and uniqueness of people, not just expanding our own influence. There is an interest in knowing other people, touching their values and traditions, and learning from them. There's almost always something to learn, even if it's not always what we might have predicted.

The personalist approach places heavy emphasis on knowing others as they are, being receptive. It looks to sharing our own values and strengths where we believe they can help, not clumsily forcing them on other people. It finds meaning in expressing concretely our respect for human life even in situations where there doesn't seem to be anything to gain, except the opportunity to express positive values in a world that would be less meaningful without our efforts.

Conclusion

This chapter puts us close to the end of the book. All that remains is the discussion of the case studies. But it's the authors' hope that this chapter also represents a beginning—a beginning of the reader's deeper personal involvement with ethical problems and their best human solutions. Since the process of personal ethics really begins with private reflection, we'd like to use this time to offer a few reflections of our own. In the Introduction, we mentioned that healing is a special kind of profession. We spoke of health care as a privilege. This is a good place to begin.

THE SPECIAL NATURE OF HEALTH CARE

For most of us, the motives that pushed us to become healers were strong and worthwhile. We wanted to develop personal skills that reinforced the best qualities we found in ourselves. We were more interested in people than in science or money. The healing professions are one of the best places to pursue this kind of inner growth. Unfortunately, as we've seen, distractions are frequent and powerful. It's easy to lose track of what were once clear and positive goals. Recentering our attention on fundamentals can be essential to our work.

What really makes healing different from other occupations? What makes it "special?" Most important is the depth of involvement that it allows in the lives of others. Healers routinely deal with the most private and sensitive of human problems. Outside the healing role, this kind of involvement might be considered meddlesome; but in a professional context, it's part of a job well done.

The healer's calling, then, can be an opportunity, an invitation, to be with people at critical times in their lives. Even before a crisis comes up, the invitation can still be there: "If I need help, I know I can turn to you." It's this invitation that provides the basis for the healing relationship. But it's important to remember that we don't really invite ourselves in—the call to personal relationship isn't a right that is ours because we've spent years preparing for it. The invitation really comes from our patients: until they open the door, the relationship can't begin. This invitation is a very personal one. It isn't based just on technical expertise or training; it's founded on a confidence in us as individuals. That's why a technical error can usually be overlooked or forgiven, but a lapse of concern often can't be. It's finally this confidence that makes our work a privilege.

Sometimes patients sense this privilege even more clearly than we do. That's why their expectations can be so high; it's also part of the reason that the health care system is in such a state of flux. Patients balk at impersonal, mechanical health care—and they should.

Healing professionals *should* be experts at achieving strong and meaningful personal relationships with others. They *should* be experts at human relationship. Unfortunately, much of our training takes the willingness to get involved for granted—so much so that we sometimes overlook it, too.

Ethics really makes sense in this kind of setting. It rounds out the knowledge we need for working with people as people, not just as biological organisms. It helps us find meaningful answers to problems we may never have encountered before. It helps us succeed.

Ethics is sometimes presented as a collection of abstract questions or issues (e.g., death and dying, patients' rights, resource allocation, and so on). But having neat, logical answers to general questions isn't really the goal of health care ethics. Meeting the needs of our patients is.

MEETING THE NEEDS OF THOSE WHO ARE ILL

What legitimate expectations do patients have of their healers? First, they expect us to be competent. They presume that we know how to do our technical job in an adequate way. Since this is the focus of most of our formal training, this is an expectation with which most of us are fairly comfortable.

Second, patients expect our respect. They want to be seen as unique individuals deserving of our esteem, and worthy of their own. Even the patient who's profoundly depressed, whose self-esteem is nearly gone, resents being treated like a number, an anonymous problem to be labeled, treated, and put aside.

Third, patients expect personal involvement and concern from their healers. They want to sense that their problems matter to us. They want us to talk with them, not at them. They want us to be there when they need us.

Fourth, they expect answers that work. They want us to approach their problems with cleverness and creativity. They want to know that, even when their situation is unusual, they can get help that is right for them and meets their needs. They expect results.

These last three expectations may seem like more than we bargained for. We're often expected to be more sensitive than average. We're expected to respond to subtle clues. Is this unreasonable? Probably not. Is it difficult? In the midst of a busy day's work, it certainly can be. But excuses won't let us escape the high standards to which we profess. This is where ethics comes in.

Ethics helps us attend to the deeper human part of our job. It keeps us from being mechanical, from missing the forest for the trees. It can keep us oriented toward quality, rather than just toward technical correctness. In the long run, it's really this feature, the focus on excellence, that separates the memorable healer from the merely adequate one.

MEETING OUR OWN NEEDS

In this book we've frequently referred to the needs of our

patients. Now let's talk a little more about our own. Patients are people; but we're people, too. Healers have unique personal needs and values, and we have personal limitations. Above all, we have a need for lasting personal relationships that are meaningful and satisfying.

We've repeatedly said that ethical reasoning can help us solve practical problems. It can help us refine our abilities as healers. Looking at ethics as a purely work-related activity, however, is like saying that we live in order to eat. Ethics has a goal that is actually more important than solving practical problems: it pushes us to find meaning throughout our lives.

In fact, if we want to find a yardstick to measure our ethical success, one of the best is the quality and depth of our most deeply chosen personal relationships. If we see those relationships growing and maturing, it's a sure bet that we're on the right inner course.

And so, it's important to remind ourselves that our families are people, too. Their value can easily be taken for granted, but our reflection should save us from that mistake. If our interest in ethics is balanced, then the relationships we've chosen for a lifetime will be kept near the surface of our attention, and those relationships will deepen and mature. But the results aren't automatic. Just as our relationships with our patients demand focused attention and concern, our relationships at home require constant tending. These relationships have to grow to survive. In order to grow, they need patience, support, and understanding. They need to be nourished with the confidence that they will work, in spite of any obstacle that could arise.

Luckily, the skills we need to reach our patients are the same ones we need to reach those we've chosen to stand by for a lifetime: listening, communicating clearly, and a sense of humor. In fact, what we do for a living should really enhance our personal lives, since it builds skills that are important to us outside our work.

It's easy to miss this connection. We'll miss it if we focus our skills on ethical sprinting, and forget about long distance running. We'll miss it if we mentally carry our work with us wherever we go. In fact, doing that, we risk going stale, running out of energy, and failing in our work as well.

We've all met excellent healers who can't seem to keep their personal lives in order. What's going wrong? It's natural for all of us to spend our efforts where we find the easiest rewards; but it's a huge mistake to neglect our larger commitments because they aren't easy. If our ethical reflections seem to fit into our role as healer, but be out of place elsewhere, then it's time to rethink.

It takes work to strengthen these relationships. In many ways, these lifetime commitments are the most difficult relationships we ever take on. But they are also the most rewarding, and the most deserving of our efforts. Although the work may not be easy, the payoffs are usually large and lasting.

Finally, our co-workers are people. They deserve our respect and support. They have complicated and unique needs that can only be met by approaching them as individuals. As we improve our ethical skills, we should see our relationships with them deepen and become more substantial.

Here again, it's easy to become distracted by the endless paperwork punctuated by the repetitive crises. It's easy to forget how important the health of the group is in the battle against illness. It's easy to forget that those who work with us are just as unique and valuable as our patients.

All of our deeper relationships are chosen and rechosen by us. They challenge us. They touch our inner freedom and promise. They help us define who we are and what we want to be. They help us chart our course. Ethics is something we can use to help us protect and enrich these relationships. In the long run, we "do" ethics for ourselves.

THE ROLE OF THE HEALER IN ETHICS

We began this book by asking, "What can ethics add to our work as healers?" Now let's reverse that question. What do we as healers have to add to the future of ethics? Embarking on a career in health care, probably the last thing on our mind was contributing to philosophy. Most of us have no formal training in philosophy, so how can we call ourselves philosophers?

However, it's important to remember that we stand in a tradition that is rich in ethical involvement. The heritage of the healing arts is replete with examples of honest concern and selflessness. Indeed, examples of thoughtlessness or superficiality are notable by their contrast.

As members of this tradition, we share in it whether we recognize it or not. Moreover, because our patients see us as representatives of this tradition, knowing what's best in an ethical sense really is a formal part of our job. In other words, we've implicitly chosen to be ethical experts by the nature of our profession.

As the "working class" of ethics, it's important to organize and share our experience. Most of us have spent more than one sleepless night worrying over an important life decision. Most of us have agonized over our limitations, and spent long hours looking for ways to help, when our scientific tools have accomplished less than we had hoped.

These trying periods were actually times of intense reflection. We were doing ethics, as focused and directed as any that has ever been done. Although we may not feel as if our conclusions were profound, the effort itself is—it represents the deepest and most profound of human feelings, the need to help. The fruit of this work is worth sharing.

Putting these ideas together and refining them is an important job. It's important to the future of health care, and it's also important to the future of ethics. Ethics is a practical science—its theory has to do more than sound good, it has to work. And, even if our ideas do work, they can always be made stronger and more effective.

There should be a concerted, cooperative effort uniting the strengths of theory and practical experience. The healing arts can provide the consummate proving ground for ethical theory, enriching and expanding the work that is carried on in our universities. Both healers and theorists can profit from each others' experiences, but, in the end, it will be our patients who profit the most.

Appendix

CASE 1. MRS. O: THE AMBIGUOUS CODE

This lady, always quiet and retiring, has fallen on hard times. Caught in a medical system renowned for its aggressiveness, she feels helpless and alone. But she's not the only one who feels helpless.

Her physician, afraid of "breaking her spirit," can't bring himself to confront his own limitations. Her nurse, afraid of getting out of line, hesitates to get more involved. Her family, trusting that good decisions will automatically be made, waits passively in the wings.

Eventually, though, Mrs. O's nurse unstalls the situation. She asks the physician to consider a social work consultation for Mrs. O, on the pretext of arranging nursing home placement. The doctor agrees, secretly relieved to get a little help with a sticky problem. He admits that he "should have thought of that himself."

The social worker sits down to chat with Mrs. O, and receives an earfull. Even Mrs. O is a bit surprised by her own temerity. She realizes that she's not doing well, but she's less afraid of death than machinery. She discusses all of her options with the social worker, whom she's begun to trust. She finally asks that her chart be changed to "no-code" status.

Over the ensuing two weeks, she has her medical ups and downs. Eventually she amazes the entire staff by recovering enough to be transferred to a nursing home, where she lives for several months.

CASE 2. THE INNOCENT BY-STANDER: WHOSE LIFE COMES FIRST?

The staff of the emergency room realized almost at once that they couldn't conduct resuscitations on two major chest wounds at the same time. The chief trauma resident ordered the main part of the team to continue their efforts on Mr. Y, but sent a junior resident and a trauma nurse to evaluate the young woman's condition, which was grave. Major efforts were made to stabilize Mr. Y, and only minor efforts were made in behalf of the lady, who indeed turned out to be his victim. In the end, both were lost.

There was a good deal of frustration and anger on the part of the emergency room staff in the days to come. There was a general sense, particularly among the nursing staff, that more should have been done for the second victim, even if that meant backing away from Mr. Y's treatment.

In an effort to deal with this issue, two meetings were held to work through the staff's concerns. In the end, most of them accepted the idea that their social role didn't include passing judgment on the actions of others. They also came to appreciate their supportive responsibilities toward each other in facing difficult situations and moving ahead.

CASE 3. THE UNHAPPY CERCLAGE

Both of these doctors seem to recognize that "doing their best" is all that can be expected. The difference, though, is that Dr. A is able to see opportunities that Dr. B misses. Being technically up to date isn't all that we have to offer as healers.

Dr. A emphasizes his technical skills because his people skills are somewhat lacking. Although his training may be superb, and his documentation may be beyond compare, he still leaves his patients with a feeling that something's missing. And it is. What's missing is his ability to communicate his depth of involvement.

Of course, we don't share our feelings with others just to avoid legal hassles, and we don't do it so that we can have a good image. We do it because those feelings are really there, and because communicating those feelings is perfectly appropriate in the context of a personal relationship.

Dr. B's objective results may not surpass Dr. A's, but his human results almost certainly do. The job of healing reaches far beyond the surface. In this case, neither doctor was sued (or even blamed) for the outcome. But Dr. A was able to leave a family that was stronger and more complete for the experience they shared. Dr. B simply left a family that was saddened by an experience that had no meaning.

CASE 4.

Discussed in Chapter 2

CASE 5. MRS. J: THE NOT-SO-ROUTINE CERVICAL CULTURE

The fact that this is a routine case is largely what makes it an important one. In fact, most of our opportunities for excellence occur in the context of the ordinary.

We're probably going to be uncomfortable with Mrs. J's reactions, because they make us confront our own insecurities—how would we handle this kind of news ourselves? In fact, the infection itself *is* fairly insignificant, in the sense that we've found it before it has become a major physical problem.

Still, the relationship between Mrs. J and her husband has been put under the spotlight. The key here is to focus on the relationship, not the infection. Is the relationship a strong and meaningful one? If it is, then it shouldn't be sacrificed to something as abstract as a subclinical disease.

If that relationship has problems and weaknesses, as most of our relationships do, then this may be a call to strengthen the relationship before it becomes even more damaged. If there's work to be done, our attention should be directed toward doing our best.

If there's no longer a viable relationship, then that difficult fact still must be faced and dealt with. Finding a place to lay blame accomplishes very little. Finding the strength to recognize problems and work to solve them can accomplish a lot.

CASE 6. MRS. C: THE ENDLESS VENTILATOR

Sometimes, in spite of our best intentions and efforts, things don't work out as planned. For Mrs. C, a chance to save her life was seen, and an appropriate attempt was made, but the situation was short-circuited by her pulmonary status. The fact that the complication wasn't anticipated really doesn't change a thing.

Now that our results have fallen short, we have to face our limitations and continue. First, we have to reassess the prognosis. Is there any real chance for Mrs. C to get off the machinery, or will these mechanical appendages necessarily be her lot indefinitely? If so, this is information she needs to have.

Also, we'll have to recognize the depth of our own responsibilities here. We've chosen to become involved with this lady in one of the most difficult problems she's ever come up against. Now that things aren't going so well, we can't just tell ourselves that it's "her problem."

We also have to ask ourselves the obvious question, "Should the ventilator be continued when it doesn't seem to be accomplishing what it was intended for—namely, temporary life support?" In the end, we're really asking ourselves whether we can help Mrs. C find a meaningful life in the midst of the suctioning and needle-sticks. The answer to that question will depend on Mrs. C's inner resources and on our own resourcefulness in helping her.

One thing we *don't* need to ask ourselves is, "Would I want to live like that?" Our job isn't to decide *for* Mrs. C, but to work with her to make the most mature decisions in the context of her own abilities and potential. Participating in this decision may be a privilege, but it's not going to be easy.

In the actual case, Mrs. C realized that she really didn't know what she was getting into when she signed the surgical permit. When the procedure was explained to her, her imagination was fixed solidly on a successful outcome.

Now she realizes that her situation is very much at odds with what she believes is right for people in general, and for herself in particular. The dialogue between her and her care-givers was a slow one, but one that helped the staff understand their own feelings better as well.

In the end, Mrs. C's two daughters were at her bedside while she was made comfortable with medication, and the ventilator was turned off. There was a general sense that everything was done to help her, and that she had given much back to her care-givers and family in her final days.

CASE 7. MR. L: THE EMPTY CODE

Mr. L wants us to do something that we don't want to do. That, in itself, isn't of much significance. The bigger problem is that what he wants will not only do him no good, but it will do violence to those around him. It's easy enough to write an order which flatly states, "full code," but quite another to do the dirty work. In this case the nursing staff is justifiably angry at being forced to participate in a macabre performance.

We can't make up our minds about what's right to do until we know a little more about Mr. L. Why is he so irrationally set on having everything done? If we talk to him a little further, we may find a good reason. Perhaps he's doing whatever he can to stay alive "until Friday, when my son gets here from Albuquerque." Then again, maybe his values are so weak that he doesn't really care about anyone else's feelings or needs. This isn't the kind of information we can infer—we have to *know*. This means spending a little time with Mr. L, whether we really can "spare the time" or not.

In this case, Mr. L had essentially alienated himself from every significant person in his life. The only relationship left was the one he had with himself, which was indeed shallow. On the basis of these values, it wasn't alright to drag everyone else down in his behalf.

Although efforts to help Mr. L do better in his final days weren't likely to succeed, that goal was pursued. Regular attempts were made to uncover deeper strengths, so that he could accept his situation and grow with it. On each occasion, Mr. L simply changed the subject.

In the end, a major effort was made to "tune" Mr. L so that he could be transferred to a nursing home. This seemed to meet with his plan for "getting better," while removing the nursing staff from a very demoralizing situation. On the third night in the nursing home, Mr. L died with little warning.

CASE 8. MR. D: SOCIAL SURGERY

In this case there seems to be a few hidden problems. Why does Mrs. D seem so intent on "doing something," when there's so little chance of success? Although it might seem to her as if she's fighting to save her husband, to some of the staff it seems more as if she's trying to punish him. Is she afraid of being alone? Are there personal or legal matters that require his attention?

What makes this case particularly difficult is that there are so few people who know Mr. D. It's critical that we learn more about him, his values, and his previous life choices. Are there children whom we could contact? Will close friends show up to visit, people who might have known him for years? Unfortunately, there were no other relatives and no close friends who were accessible.

In the end, one of the surgeons agreed to operate on Mr. D. The surgery went fairly smoothly, but there were multiple postoperative complications. He died on the second day after surgery.

In an ethical sense, though, that was just the beginning. Mrs. D has singled herself out as a person in need of help, of healing. Trying to stay in touch with her, to be available to help with her loss, was really the only productive thing the professional team had to offer. These efforts were made, but only Mrs. D would ever know if this work was important to her, since she continued to reveal very little about her feelings.

CASE 9. MR. K: "I DON'T WANT TO KNOW"

This case occurred before widespread informed consent for AIDS testing was instituted. Today, this particular problem might not stretch our imaginations, but ones like it still come up regularly. In the long run, waiting for the law to catch up to our problems simply isn't practical—we really can't escape the need to develop our own ethical judgment, or the fact that ultimately we alone are responsible for our personal choices.

The nurse in this case felt very strongly that ordering a test as emotionally sensitive as an AIDS test should be done only with the patient's knowledge. When the test returned positive, he was faced with the same issue again, but the tables were turned. Now the patient (instead of the surgeon) had become the "withholder of information," and the patient's partner had become the unsuspecting victim. He's found himself in the unenviable position of being the one who tells the truth for those around him. How far does this job description go?

Of course, it would have been nice if the nurse could have convinced the surgeon to inform his patients about these tests; but that approach had already failed previously, and wasn't likely to work this time either. Trying to do the surgeon's job for him, though, is a little too much to take on, and the hospital administration might have been helpful in supplying guidelines for cases like this one.

However, this still doesn't help us with the patient's boyfriend. Should we tell or not? Again, we have to ask ourselves how much responsibility we really have. In this case, the boyfriend could be expected to have a certain amount of knowledge about the spread of AIDS, and it would be reasonable to expect him to investigate the situation on his own.

What about cases where people are in grave danger, and have no way of suspecting that the danger is there? If we have this kind of knowledge, there are both legal and moral obligations to step forward. In this case, such compelling reasons don't exist. In fact, it turned out that the boyfriend had also taken the position that he "didn't want to know."

CASE 10. MR. R: A FAMILY AFFAIR

Sometimes, as in this case, we have too many questions and too little time to answer them. The disagreement among the family members here could take days to sort out; but the decisions couldn't wait.

Even if we mistrust the wife's opinion about what her husband would want, it carries a great deal of weight. Perhaps

Mr. R really wouldn't want surgery, all things being equal, but would submit to it for her sake alone. Perhaps, if we operate, he'll live to tell us that we did the wrong thing. We can't really answer these questions now.

What happened was this. Surgery was performed, and Mr. R tolerated the procedure remarkably well. Unfortunately, he failed to regain consciousness afterward. Mrs. R asked that life support be withdrawn in the week following surgery and that was done. Special efforts were made to talk further with her and to reassure her that her choices were alright.

Also, time was spent with the other dissenting family members to make sure that they had ample opportunities to discuss their feelings. They were encouraged to give support to Mrs. R just as their father would have wanted them to. In the end, the family seemed to be brought together by an issue that had initially divided them.

CASE 11. MRS. T: A STROKE OF BAD LUCK

This is a common type of case. Mrs. T seems to have lost the potential for meaningful thought, and we don't have the means to restore it. Since she's breathing on her own, however, no unusual care is needed to sustain her.

Still, the fact that her tube feedings have no real chance of restoring her human faculties makes them effectively "extraordinary." The fact that these feedings are fairly easy to do doesn't automatically justify their use. Some will argue that withdrawing this type of basic support will cause her deep physical discomfort which we can't verify. Actually, we have perfectly good mechanisms for alleviating discomfort, even if we withhold fluids.

In fact, keeping Mrs. T alive with nothing to live for speaks more to our own anxiety about death than our respect for life. It also highlights our own insecurity about our technical limitations.

In this case, special efforts were made to identify family or loved ones, so that they could be allowed to "say good-bye." There turned out to be no one to contact, though. An informal meeting of the nursing staff was called to discuss the situation. There turned out to be a surprising uniformity of support for the idea of allowing Mrs. T to die peacefully. Her nasogastric feedings were discontinued, she was kept comfortable with medication, and died two nights later.

CASE 12. BABY S: "GOD'S WILL BE DONE"

Through our surgical intervention, we have an excellent chance to allow Baby S to live many years. Although she might never earn a college degree, she will probably be very capable of appreciating life and finding meaning in her relationships. In fact, looking at our nuclear arsenal, one has to wonder if intelligence is the most worthwhile of human characteristics.

Sacrificing this child would be wrong. Discussions about "God's will" in matters such as this one really lead nowhere. Actually, each of us has limitations, but ascribing them to God only excuses us from trying to grow and be better than we presently are. This is not what ethics is about.

In this case, the parents are looking for some way to avoid shouldering a heavy burden that has come their way. The best way to help with their problem is to provide more shoulders to carry the load. All available personal and social resources should be used to help them meet this unanticipated problem. Their limitations, like their child's, can't be wished away.

Surgery was performed and the child did very well. The parents came to realize that having a "defective" child was nothing to be ashamed of—indeed, it turned out to be an opportunity to demonstrate their love in an extraordinary way. They went on to have three more normal children, and found that their Down's child contributed greatly to their family.

CASE 13. MRS. N: ABORTION IN ELEPHANT BUTTE

In this case, the physician was strongly opposed to abortion for moral reasons, but he also felt committed to help his patient. He didn't consider it sufficient "help" simply to inform her that abortion is wrong.

He looked into social support services, but they were pathetically lacking in this rural community. He brought up the idea of adoption, and even went so far as to consider adopting the child himself. Unfortunately, the realities of the situation were against that: the husband wouldn't have allowed it.

The possibility of leaving her husband was explored, but Mrs. N wasn't able to face that prospect. She had no other familial support, and continued to hope that she could help him deal with his addiction to alcohol. She repeatedly spoke of his good qualities, and her sense of commitment to him.

In the end, having looked at, and rejected, all the other possibilities, the physician did perform the abortion. This was done with great regret, as well as a little anger at the circumstances that seemed to require it. Special attention was directed toward Mr. N, who eventually made surprising progress in dealing with his alcoholism. He never learned of the abortion or the struggle his wife underwent in this case.

CASE 14. TOM G: DEATH WITH DIGNITY

Everything was handled in this case in a particularly excellent manner. Meetings were arranged for Tom's mother with a social worker, a minister, and a psychologist—none of whom were able to establish rapport with her. Every effort was made to help her deal with the problem. Even so, she stood her ground.

In fact, she stood by, arms folded, while Tom twice underwent difficult resuscitation. The third time Tom's heart stopped, his mother was at dinner, and, although resuscitation was begun, it was "unsuccessful." To the last, Tom's mother believed that she had done the right thing.

The ICU staff was highly disrupted by this case. They felt as if they had done the wrong thing, as if they had abused the very patient they had become so fond of. It took two group meetings with a psychologist to begin to work through these feelings, to help the team begin to function as a unit again.

In retrospect, the one resource that was overlooked, sadly, was Tom himself. Although there was an effort to *use* him to change his mother's mind, he wasn't involved in the problem in a really meaningful way. He was kept at a distance from his mother, instead of being allowed to help her. In the end, he remained the object of everyone's concern, but had only a peripheral part in the drama itself.

CASE 15. MR. P: WHAT'S REALLY GOING ON HERE?

The physicians in this case were ready to give up on Mr. P—perhaps a little too soon. Several critical tests had not been performed, and so the prognosis was still a bit unclear. His rapidly deteriorating course certainly wasn't a good sign, but there were just too many loose ends.

There was a sharp division among the resident physicians in this case. On one hand, some of them wanted to continue aggressive treatment indefinitely, apparently hoping that something would somehow "turn up." On the other hand, some wanted to just "pull the plug" and move on. Neither side seemed able to appreciate the other's point of view. Mr. P didn't give any sign that he cared who won this debate.

Because a spinal tap hadn't been performed, and because blood cultures were taken only after antibiotics had been begun, the antibiotics were first withdrawn. After two days, there was no evidence that an occult infection was present. Since the other potential causes of coma were irreversible, it was clear that no other treatable problems were present. Ventilator support was withdrawn, and Mr. P died.

The rift between the house-staff still needed to be mended, though. A case conference was held, and the case was discussed at length. Two of the residents, particularly involved in the case, came forward later to talk out their concerns. Although never setting out to be a teacher, Mr. P proved to be a source of learning for several of the young physicians.

CASE 16. MR. H: A GOOD DAY TO DIE

In itself, this wouldn't be a particularly difficult case, except that everyone involved seems to have a different idea of what should be done. A storm is brewing, and poor Mr. H is at its center.

What's most important here is to make sure that the damage caused by the disease isn't greater than it has to be. Even if we decide that his daughter is "wrong" in demanding surgery, we have to accept the fact that she's a very important person to Mr. H, and that her feelings and needs really do matter. Our responsibilities to Mr. H extend to those who are significant to him. In the context of a responsible personal relationship, it isn't always up to us to pick and choose.

There are other problems as well. There are staff members who are becoming ill because of their inability to agree on what's right for Mr. B. The only reason they are having problems with his case is because they *care*. This isn't a weakness, but a human problem brought about by Mr. B's physical condition. Helping to heal the staff can be an important and valuable job, if we're up to it.

In this case, the staff members made a special effort to work in the family's behalf, rather than to push stubbornly for the choices they imagined they would have made themselves. They made an extra effort to remain receptive to the daughter's needs, even though they had some emotional misgivings toward her opinions.

In the end, Mr. H agreed to undergo the chemotherapy, but not the surgery. His daughter supported his decision. Unfortunately, his course was a rapidly downhill one, which gave the chemotherapy very little chance to work. Much to the staff's surprise, the daughter sent a gift to the ward after his funeral, thanking them for their caring and support.

CASE 17. MRS. V: A NON-LIVING WILL

The staff realized that Mrs. V really had very little idea of what she was doing when she signed the living will. They documented their impressions and moved on. Chemotherapy was begun and there was an initial positive response. About two weeks into her treatment, though, the tumor began to grow rapidly.

In keeping with her perceived wishes, a tracheostomy was scheduled, but she died before this was able to be carried out. Mr. V was upset at the outcome, but soon expressed relief that his wife was no longer suffering, and that she was now finally at peace.

CASE 18. MRS. M: ENOUGH IS ENOUGH

In this case, there was a feeling among some of the staff members that Mrs. M was making a rational decision and that it should be supported. The technician who received the call, though, felt as if she knew Mrs. M better than that. She called Mrs. M back a short while later, and asked if she could visit Mrs. M at home after work. Mrs. M agreed.

In their conversation, several significant facts came out, confirming the technician's suspicions that there was more going on than was apparent on the surface. She became convinced that Mrs. M was much too upset over a number of family problems to make such a serious life decision.

She asked Mrs. M to give her problems just one more week's try. Again, Mrs. M agreed, although a little reluctantly. Over the ensuing week, Mrs. M was able to gain a much deeper insight into her feelings. She eventually carried through with her treatment for nearly a year, when she died of complications of her disease.

CASE 19. GARY: THERAPY OR TORTURE?

In the actual case, the oncologist turned out to be an extraordinarily difficult person to know. His motivation in this treatment reversal remained a mystery. Although there was never any doubt that he was doing what he thought was best for Gary, it wasn't clear whether he was fooling himself out of personal weakness.

Gary tolerated the new chemotherapy remarkably well, but he didn't respond physically. The staff worked especially hard to keep his spirits up, and they did a remarkably good job. Gary didn't do well with his leukemia, but he certainly did well with his illness. The staff was very much saddened when he died, but they were relieved that his problems had ended.

Even though the staff was satisfied that they had done all they could for Gary, they still felt a great sense of loss and inadequacy for not being able to save him. They held two meetings with a staff psychologist to work out their problems so that they wouldn't be crippled by their loss. They eventually purchased a special plaque in honor of Gary, and hung it in a prominent place in the pediatric oncology wing.

Bibliography

WORKS OF GENERAL INTEREST

Abrams, Morris B. et al. *Deciding to Forego Life-Sustaining Treatment*. Washington D.C.: President's Commission for the Study of Ethical Problems in Medicine and Biomedical and Behavioral Research, 1983.

———. *Splicing Life*. Washington D.C.: President's Commission for the Study of Ethical Problems in Medicine and Biomedical and Behavioral Research, 1982.

Arras, John and Hunt, Robert. *Ethical Issues in Modern Medicine*. Palo Alto, Calif.: Mayfield Publishing Company, 1983.

Ashley, Benedict M. and O'Rourke, Kevin D. *Health Care Ethics, A Theological Analysis*. St. Louis: The Catholic Health Association of the United States, 1982.

Fromm, Erich. *Man for Himself*. New York: Rinehart and Co, 1947.

Veatch, Robert M. *Case Studies in Medical Ethics*. Cambridge, Mass.: Harvard University Press, 1977.

DEONTOLOGY

Beauchamp, Tom L. and Childress, James F. *Principles of Biomedical Ethics*. New York: Oxford University Press, 1983.

Kant, Immanuel. *Critique of Practical Reason*. Chicago: Encyclopaedia Britannica, 1955.

UTILITARIANISM

Mill, John Stuart. *Utilitarianism*. New York: The Liberal Arts Press, 1953.

CONTRACT THEORY

Rawls, John. *A Theory of Justice*. Cambridge, Mass.: Belknap Press, 1971.
Veatch, Robert M. *A Theory of Medical Ethics*. New York: Basic Books, 1981.

SITUATION ETHICS

Fletcher, Josef F. *Situation Ethics*. Philadelphia: Westminster Press, 1966.

VIRTUE THEORY

Aristotle. *Nicomachean Ethics*. Indianapolis: Bobbs-Merrill Educational Publishing, 1983.
MacIntyre, Alasdair. *After Virtue: A Study in Moral Theory*. Notre Dame: University of Notre Dame Press, 1981.

PERSONALISM

Berdyaev, Nicolas. *The Destiny of Man*. New York: Harper and Row, 1960.
Mounier, Emmanuel. *Personalism*. London: Routledge and Kegan Paul, 1952.
Weiss, Paul. *Privacy*. Carbondale: Southern Illinois University Press, 1983.
————. *You, I, and the Others*. Carbondale: Southern Illinois University Press, 1980.

Index

AIDS, 55
abortion, 53–54, 87–89, 111–12
Aristotle, 72
autonomy, 42, 53, 65

beneficence, 42, 65
business aspects of health care, 10–12

Categorical Imperative, 65
choices, reflective, 22–23
coercion, 46
commercialism, 108
communication, 78, 86, 122
competence, 45
confidentiality, 54–56
conflicts of responsibility, 48, 57–58, 101
consequentialism, 68–70
consumerism, 31
contract theory, 67–68
contracts, 45
cost containment, 11
cost/benefit, 44
curing or caring, 30

death, 37, 113; definition of, 47
decision making, 116
defective infants, 59–60, 112–13
deontology, 64–67
disease, 28–30

documentation, 9
duties, absolute, 65
duties, relative, 65–66

eclecticism, 73
economics, 10–12
education, 112, 115
ethics, 4; and decision making, 37; definition of, 18–21, 25; goals of, 12, 123; and health care, 36, 121; and meaning, 36; social, 5–7, 44, 58–59, 105–18
euthanasia, 52–53, 87–89, 113–15
evil, 87
excellence, 12–13
extraordinary means, 48, 115–16

Fletcher, Josef, 70
following through, 102–3
freedom, 81, 118

genetic engineering, 60–61

Harvard Criteria, 47
healing, 32–34
health care education, 12
human experimentation, 47, 61
human uniqueness, 77

illness, 33, 34

illness v. disease, 28–30, 91,
95–96
impartiality, 69
informed consent, 46
institutional review boards
(IRBs), 47–48
issues, personal v. social, 107

judgmentalism, 16, 84
justice, 43, 65, 67

Kantianism, 42–43, 64–67

law, 7–10, 17, 107
law, conflict with, 71
listening, 86
living will, 45, 98

malpractice, 7–10
meaning, 25, 76, 112, 114; definition of, 19
meaning of relationship, 76
Mounier, Emmanuel, 23

obligation, social, 85
openness, 21, 84, 93, 118
ordinary means, 48, 115–16
organ transplantation, 59

paternalism, 44–45
person, definition of, 79–83, 111,
112, 114
personalism, 75
philosophy, 19, 123
politics, 105–18
principles: ethical, 42–43, 64;
personal, 17, 89
prognosis of disease, 94

promise, human, 81

quality as goal of health care,
12–13

Rawls, John, 67
reflection, 22–23, 37, 77, 93
relationship: and health care,
120, 122; personal, 76, 83–85,
97–99, 114
resource allocation, 58–59
respect for the human person,
76, 93, 110, 117, 121
responsibility, global, 116–18
responsibility, personal, 85, 114
resuscitation, 3
right to die, 64
rules of conduct, 16

scientific model, 4, 12, 28
self-awareness, 80
situation ethics, 70–71

technology: personal issues, 2–5,
32; social issues, 5–7
trust, 84
truth telling, 56

utilitarianism, 68–70

values, 25, 35, 83, 110; definition
of, 20; health care, 27, 30–32;
negative and positive, 20–21
virtue theory, 71–73
vulnerability, 84–85

Weiss, Paul, 83, 98
whistle-blowing, 48
withdrawal of support, 94

ABOUT THE AUTHORS

WILLIAM dePENDER is a practicing physician in Seattle, Washington. He received his B.A. in philosophy from Gonzaga University in Spokane, and his M.D. from the University of Washington. His work experience includes three years at one of the nation's largest indigent care institutions, Charity Hospital of New Orleans; two years on the Navajo reservation at Fort Defiance, Arizona; and four years of urban private practice in Seattle.

In 1984 he spent a year as visiting scholar at the Kennedy Institute of Ethics in Washington, D.C., studying under the direction of Dr. Edmund Pellegrino, one of this country's foremost health care ethicists. Dr. dePender has continued his involvement in ethics through teaching in the graduate school of Seattle University, and through lecturing in the Seattle area.

WANDA IKEDA-CHANDLER earned her Bachelor of Science degree in Nursing from the University of Washington. She has ten years of direct patient care experience as an emergency room nurse in major urban trauma centers. She is currently nurse-manager of the Emergency Department and the Emergency Medical Services at the Oxford-Lafayette Medical Center in Oxford, Mississippi.